PRESCRIPTION: MEDICIDE

DR. JACK

KEVORKIAN

BY THE
INVENTOR OF THE
CONTROVERSIAL
"SUICIDE MACHINE"

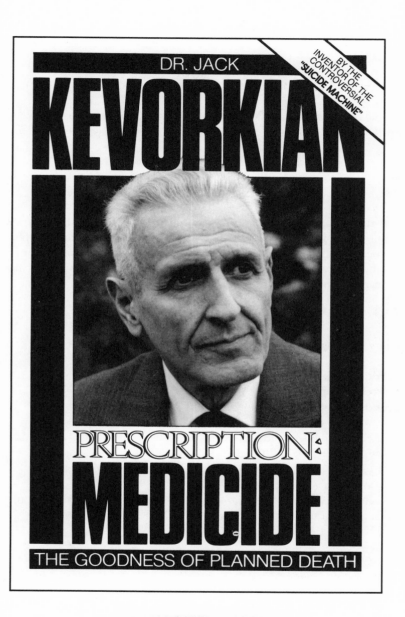

PRESCRIPTION
MEDICIDE

THE GOODNESS OF PLANNED DEATH

PROMETHEUS BOOKS
BUFFALO, NEW YORK

Published 1991 by Prometheus Books

editorial offices located at 700 East Amherst Street, Buffalo, New York 14215; distribution facilities at 59 John Glenn Drive, Amherst, New York 14228.

95 94 93 92 91   5 4 3 2 1

Library of Congress Cataloging-in-Publication Data

Kevorkian, Jack.
    Prescription—medicide : the goodness of planned death / Jack Kevorkian.—1st ed.
        p.   cm.
    Includes bibliographical references and index.
    ISBN 0-87975-677-2 (cloth)
    1. Euthanasia. 2. Right to die. 3. Suicide. 4. Executions and executioners. 5. Organ donors. I. Title.
    [DNLM: 1. Ethics, Medical—popular works. 2. Euthanasia—popular works. 3. Right to Die—popular works. W 50 K43p]
R726.K48   1991
179'.7—dc20
DNLM/DLC
for Library of Congress   89-92751

Printed on acid-free paper in the United States of America

To
those enlightened doctors
in
ancient Hellenistic Alexandria
and
medieval Cilician Armenia

They dared to do what is right

Acknowledgments

I thank Hugh Wray McCann both for his encouragement and for his proofreading; Ms. Margo Janus for proofreading and helping to prepare the manuscript; and Steven L. Mitchell, my editor at Prometheus Books, for his invaluable assistance.

Contents

1

Retribution on the 13th of July

"We're ready now."

It seemed like an almost obscene interruption by an irrelevant voice—an utterance of strained indifference, feigned sympathy, and scornful relief. The vacuous gaze of the emotionally drained twenty-eight-year-old man drifts toward the source of the interruption. It was a guard merely doing his duty.

"Yea, though I walk through . . . ." The 23rd Psalm was also interrupted, and the chaplain's reverent droning stops abruptly. He gently closes the Good Book over an index finger, lowers it to his side, and glances at his wristwatch. It is exactly 11:45 P.M. "The time has come, my son"; he almost whispers in as gentle a tone as he can muster. The mute convict slowly rises from the edge of a narrow cot fastened to the bare wall of his cell on Louisiana's death row.

For what must have seemed like eons the three stand there—
the inmate, the chaplain, and the slightly nervous guard—but it was
only a matter of seconds. The convict shifts his gaze from the chaplain
to the guard's face—but piercing far beyond it to dissolve in rapid,
disjointed images of a bungled bank robbery, futile kidnapping of
two hostages, and their senselessly brutal murder when ransom demands were ignored. These flash through the inmate's panic-stricken
mind like an unedited movie of assorted outtakes, while with the
slow, measured stride of an automaton he dutifully trails the guard
out of his last earthly residence. Behind him saunters the chaplain,
who has resumed his monotonous scriptural recitation.

Jumbled thoughts and jumbled images. "Is there a God? If there
is, then woe is me! If not, then what? Am I on the verge of rotting
to nothing but scaly bones to be dug up and fondly analyzed by some
sort of archaeologist a million years from now? Or, maybe to just
dissolve away to nothing in the earth's magma? Where am I going
to go in a minute or two? And why?"

The young man's deceptively tranquil physique is nothing other
than a crucible of wrenching seismic clashes among all kinds of notions of good and bad, life and death. "How did this all happen?
If only I had listened to my old man and stayed in school. God,
how I wish I could have become that architect or engineer I always
dreamed of being as a kid. What terrific ideas I had for new buildings
and bridges. Then there was that chance to join the Peace Corps.
Why didn't I take it? Maybe that could have kept me from sinking
to this. Why? Why?"

The solemn procession slowly makes its way into the execution
chamber. As though in a trance the doomed man is oblivious of everything—until he confronts directly the last place on earth he will sit
while still alive.

There it is, in all its mocking terror: the notorious chair he had
read and heard so much about. A crude but sturdy thing of solid
oak with heavy leather straps dangling by its sides like the sinuous
tentacles of an ogre anxious to seize and devour him. Even the coarse

folds in the rubber mask slung over a post of the backrest seem to taunt him with a sardonic smile.

His frantic eyes scan the thickly insulated cables connecting the ogre like an umbilical cord to a wall panel adorned with a bewildering array of dials, knobs, and switches. And as the head-plate electrode devours his scalp like the maw of that ogre, he struggles valiantly—without much success—to reassure himself that all of this is merely an invention of the human mind in the hope that it will somehow ease the expunging of his life demanded by a debtor society.

The convict's white-hot brain crackles with seemingly unanswerable questions. "Is this just a bad dream, or is it for real? Are my wrists and ankles really being fettered to this ugly thing, or is it just my tortured imagination? And how about all those gawkers in the gallery; are they real, too? Or, will this whole sordid mess disappear in a flash when the jolt shocks me awake from this nightmare?"

All eyes focus on the large clock on the wall. It's now two minutes before midnight. The telephone rings once, twice, three times. The warden puts the receiver to his ear, listens for about ten seconds, then hangs up. His dour countenance conveys an unspoken message: no reprieve. The execution will proceed without delay.

There is stony silence in the spectator gallery. The executioner is given a signal as the second hand of the clock sweeps through the final half minute to exactly midnight.

Suddenly 2,000 volts drive eight death-dealing amperes at the speed of light through the heavy cables on the electrodes on the head-cap. At the same time a surge of ethereal power engulfs the spectator gallery to evince scattered gasps of shocked fascination. A few lower jaws involuntarily drop in dumb, open-mouthed reaction to a gruesome first experience. Here and there, offended eyes shut out the sight of it completely, or only half-heartedly with heads askance or bowed. Inured souls gaze fixedly and without emotion at what they've seen before.

It isn't every day that one sees a human body turned into a high tension line. The current surges through the convict's head and body to complete the circuit at the electrode connected above the right ankle. A tiny puff of steam and smoke wafting from beneath the reverberating face-mask shows that the circuit is complete. It heralds physiological and anatomical cataclysm, biological electrochemical chaos, tremendous heat, and coagulation of protoplasm.

The mask only partially hides grotesque grimaces that exaggerate and even belie sensibility, for a cooking brain no longer regulates what is perceived and what the response will be. Muscles jerk violently and arms and legs strain at their bonds as the voltage is reduced to 500 volts for thirty seconds.

Then back up to 2,000 volts. Wrists and ankles curl rigid, with fingers and toes tightly flexed. Again down to 500 volts, and once more up to 2,000. Only a single thought now dominates the agitated minds in the gallery: "Enough! That's enough!" The power is switched off at one minute and twenty-seven seconds after midnight.

The spastic body relaxes slightly. A medical doctor adjusts the ear-pieces of his stethoscope and approaches the motionless form in the warm chair, bares the left chest, and places the scope's bell on the hot skin over the heart. There is no sign of breathing. Bent forward and staring blindly at the floor, the doctor listens searchingly over the precordial area.* After about one minute his face manifests perplexed disbelief. The heart is still beating faintly!

Consternation ripples through the awe-struck gallery. A benumbed reporter whispers to a colleague, "My God, what a horrendous mess. And so unnecessary. Now they're going to have to repeat the damned horror show with literal overkill! Don't they know that simple 100 volt house current with the man's feet in a bucket of water will do the trick fast, sure, and neat?" The listener nods almost imperceptibly without turning, as though himself stunned into near paralysis.

It is eight minutes after midnight when the executioner throws the switch for the second time.

The inmate's body reacts with milder spasms. After all, his tissue proteins already are partly clotted, energy stores used up, and enzymes destroyed. Parts of the exposed skin now show the splotchy,

---

*The area over the heart.

coarse purple-red to yellow-tan effect of the continued electrical assault. Fragile areas around the head electrodes ooze streaks of magenta blood. Visually the scene can be blotted out at will, but nobody can escape the sickening, pungent stench of seared flesh beginning to permeate the chamber.

The heart had now stopped. It had to because its muscle protoplasm was coagulating, if not already thoroughly cooked. This time the doctor heard nothing through his stethoscope. Officially the recorded time of death was 00:15 on 13 July.

Observers began filing out of the gallery with relief. The reporter stopped and looked back reflectively. Guards were removing the bloody electrodes and the taut limb restraints while the medical examiner waited to take custody of the remains. A sort of qualified satisfaction passed through the reporter's mind as he turned to follow his silent colleague into the noisy press room. "Well, that's that," he mused tacitly. "The killer has paid his debt to society. It's retribution, and justice has been served."

It was seventeen minutes after midnight by the clock on the press room wall.

2

What *Really* Happened?

Hilo, Hawaii. 12 July, 08:15 P.M.

M. L., a thirty-nine-year-old wife and mother of three young daughters, turns her sleepless eyes to the window of her hospital room. Her occasional sighs express considerable pity, a bit for herself but more for her beloved family. Again today there was no good news from her doctor. Neither can a sympathetic hospital staff offer more than trite words of encouragement to their very depressed patient whose condition is slipping out of control.

For several years now M. L. has been undergoing kidney dialysis because of progressive renal failure as a result of glomerulonephritis (formerly better known as Bright's disease).*At first the dire con-

---

*Chronic inflammation of the kidneys.

sequences of the disease were pretty much held in check by regulating salt and protein in the diet and through dialysis twice a week on the artificial kidney in her home. In time the dialysis had to be increased to three times a week. Furthermore, the feared complication of hypertension (high blood pressure) required that she begin taking antihypertensive medication.

During the past several months the forearm fistula used for needle connections for tubes directing blood flow between her and the machine had begun to show signs of obstructive tissue growth and clotting. Anemia also made frequent blood transfusions necessary, and that exposed her to the serious risk of hepatitis. Worst of all her depression was rapidly deepening. The situation called for immediate hospitalization.

M. L.'s fortitude had been exhausted. She now had no other choice. A kidney transplant would be her only option. The decision was easy for her and her family. Implementing it was another matter.

For several weeks now M. L.'s name has been on the waiting list of needy recipients being processed through the computerized nationwide organ procurement and matching network. Initial optimism faded as weeks passed without the eagerly anticipated telephone call announcing the computer's donor match. If she only knew exactly where her name is on that list. But then, maybe it's better that she doesn't know; benevolent ignorance keeps hope flickering. But only barely.

Yakutat, Alaska. 12 July, 09:15 P.M.

An eighteen-year-old student, Z. M., lies propped up as he reads by a light over the head of his bed on the ward of a small hospital. Two years ago he began having headaches and complained about an irksome loss of "pep" and a poor appetite accompanied by slight nausea. At the same time, he noticed occasional swelling of the ankles and a fairly constant, vague ache in both flanks. But it was the appearance of red blood in the urine which prompted a hasty visit to his doctor.

On physical examination large, soft, knobby masses were detected in both sides of the upper abdomen. Ultrasonography revealed the diagnosis: numerous destructive cysts, some very large, in both kidneys.

Z. M.'s kidney function deteriorated rapidly as his blood pressure rose to dangerous levels, necessitating aggressive drug treatment. Within several weeks he needed artificial kidney dialysis, often three times a week. Faced with the bleak prospect of a long life dependent on that machine and all the potential complications of the disease (such as hypertension with resultant stroke or heart attack, hepatitis from transfusions, urinary tract infections, and mental depression), this young man is an ideal candidate for a kidney transplant.

His name has been on the computerized network for four months now. While waiting for that telephone call from the Anchorage medical center, like M. L., he, too, keeps wondering just where his name is on that list.

Fresno, California. 12 July, 10:15 P.M.

A. W. languishes between semicoma and sleep in a private hospital room. Three years earlier the married forty-one-year-old school teacher, husband, and father of a small son and infant daughter began having vague, nonspecific symptoms: headache, poor appetite, nausea, and extreme muscle weakness. Shortly thereafter a yellowish tint appeared in the white of his eyes. Later a medical checkup revealed mild fever and more pronounced yellow-tan discoloration of the entire skin. In addition, there were bulging and irregularly tortuous veins on the abdomen; and his stool had turned pitch black.

On the second day after entering the hospital A. W. vomited a small amount of dark red blood. X-rays showed the source to be dilated veins in the esophagus. His liver was small, hard, and slightly tender. A needle biopsy of the liver yielded the conclusive answer: severe atrophic cirrhosis with extensive scarring. Most of what was left of the functioning liver tissue showed signs of impending degeneration.

The exact cause of the devastating process was obscure. A. W.

had never been a heavy or even moderate drinker. But about twelve years earlier he had a severe attack of the "flu," which his doctor thought was infectious mononucleosis. His current prognosis is not good.

It is obvious that without a liver transplant he won't last long. His name has been on the network's list for the past two weeks. Prospects seem to be dim to nil.

Denver, Colorado. 12 July, 11:15 P.M.

T. J., a thirty-two-year-old secretary, drowsily stares into the shadowy space of her semiprivate hospital room. The pillows propping her up seem to be doing little to ease the short, quick gasps of her labored breathing. Especially worrisome and annoying is the forceful, sometimes irregular thumping of her straining heart against the chest wall.

Mild symptoms began about nine months earlier. Increasing weakness, shortness of breath, and anxiety over heart palpitations caused her to seek medical help. The doctors were baffled by the nonspecific findings on physical examination. But ominous changes in the electrocardiographic (ECG) tracing convinced them that it was some kind of heart disease. Worsening of symptoms led her to seek hospitalization for definitive tests and the quick institution of therapy if called for and if possible.

An accurate diagnosis could be approximated only through a process of elimination. Two days of routine and highly sophisticated tests and procedures indicated the probability of so-called cardiomyopathy (a "sick heart muscle").

Absolute bed rest and medication did little good in controlling the increasingly frequent disturbances in heart rhythm. Weakness and shortness of breath grew worse, and several days ago signs of early heart failure appeared. Doctors know that the course of this disease is unpredictable but usually quite short and grim. In her case it has been extraordinarily rapid, and the prognosis is bad—indeed hopeless if she does not get a heart transplant soon.

Without a doubt her recent periods of insomnia are due to more than the symptoms of her disease. Where is *her* name on the computerized list?

Springfield, Illinois. 13 July, 00:15 A.M.

Fifty-four-year-old H. L. T. is comfortably seated in a reclining chair at home, watching a late-night TV movie in the company of his wife and adolescent son. His obvious distress is manifested by rapid and shallow breathing which, together with the oxygen tube in his nose, compels him to speak short, staccato-like phrases with a subdued voice. His long stretches of silence are understandable.

Many years ago H. L. T. sensed a gradual shortness of breath, sometimes with a mild, dry cough. Occasional "colds" made the coughing worse, at times accompanied by wheezing. He began losing weight, too; but it was the shortness of breath that alarmed him.

A thorough medical examination six years earlier, including X-rays and lung function studies, revealed abnormally large clear spaces, some of them huge, in both lungs; and their functional capacity was markedly diminished. The diagnosis was chronic obstructive pulmonary disease, better known as emphysema. In H. L. T.'s case the cause was unclear. He had smoked cigarettes only briefly as a youth (about half a pack a day for three years) but had given up the habit over thirty years ago. A special laboratory test now revealed that he lacked an important enzyme known to protect against the onset of this baffling disease.

Treatment has been merely supportive with oxygen, antibiotics, and bronchodilators to help control the ever worsening wheezing on prolonged exhalation of each labored breath.

Doctors have concluded that his only hope is to have a lung transplant as soon as possible. His name was added to the national waiting list for that very precious and rare item.

Wheeling, West Virginia. 13 July, 01:15 A.M.

A thin, well developed nineteen-year-old man, K. T., falls into a light sleep in a hospital bed adjusted to a near-sitting position. But bed rest and oxygen supplied by a nasal tube cannot alleviate his labored breathing. Short gasps are accompanied by marked motion of a thin chest wall coarsely corrugated by a prominent rib cage. Cadaverous skin pallor is tinged with a dusky blue of cyanosis.* His anxious face underscores constant air hunger and the hopelessness of depression.

It all started three years ago with the usual mild and vague symptoms of weakness, fatigue, and loss of appetite. About a year later he began feeling dull aches in his chest. Occasional coughs were usually dry, but at times produced yellowish discharge. His doctor prescribed treatment for bronchitis, after which the coughing disappeared for several months. When it recurred, the mucus was streaked with a small amount of blood. The doctor then admitted him to the hospital for intensive investigation.

Besides being anemic, K. T. also had significantly reduced functional capacity of the lungs. Fresh blood was detected in lung fluid. Microscopic examination of a thin needle biopsy through the thin chest wall confirmed a rare diagnosis: bleeding and deposits of blood pigment in lung tissue beginning to undergo scarring, cause unknown.

There is no specific or curative treatment. Oxygen helped his breathing, and antibiotics cleared up the bronchial infection. This allowed him to stay at home for long periods of time. But he had to be hospitalized again when he became very short of breath and a fair amount of blood was coughed up five days earlier. Supportive therapy has been continued, but it is obvious that his disease has progressed to a very dangerous stage. Doctors are sure that he won't last long.

K. T.'s name has been on the network's list for five days.

---

*Skin color change due to poor circulation and lack of oxygen in the blood.

Death row, Louisiana. 12 July, 11:30 P.M.

"It's stupid and crazy! It's wrong! It's downright cruel!" The seated condemned man's angry eyes glare at the chaplain. "Nobody listens to me. Nobody cares. My God, nobody even cares!" And with a furious mixture of anger and contempt, he adds, "Maybe *you'll* listen. Maybe *you* can do something before it's too late."

A desperate glimmer of hope flashes from the inmate's eyes. He snatches some wrinkled papers off his cot, springs to his feet, and thrusts them into the chaplain's hands. "Here, look at these. Just look at the cowardly buck-passing. No damn guts. Look here—see how they all run for cover, these phony do-gooders!"

The chaplain takes three letters from the inmate's trembling hand and begins to scan them quickly.

"Dear Sir: I have your recent letter regarding your wish to have organs taken for transplantation to needy patients when you are executed. This is certainly a noble and humanitarian gesture by you. But I cannot approve your request. Even if you resort to court action, the Corrections Department would still oppose your request because of the dangerous legal implications and precedents. Respectfully, (signed by the Commissioner.)"

Gently biting his lower lip, the chaplain subtly displays a vague sense of disquieting incredulity rippling through his mind as he shuffles to the next letter.

"Dear Sir: Our chief of transplant surgery asked me to respond to your recent letter to him. Your present situation makes such donation of organs impossible under the current laws of this state. And, as far as we know, no other state has permitted donation under such circumstances. However, you are certainly to be commended for your humanitarian gesture. Sincerely, (signed by the administrator of the University Medical Center)."

Now deeply reflective, the chaplain seems to be immersed in a tacit soliloquy as he pulls out the third and last letter.

"Dear Sir: Your recent letter shows great depth of feeling, and your desire to help others is very commendable. However, even though I applaud your desire to have another person benefit from your life, I cannot approve donation of your organs. The state is required, by law, to maintain you as an inmate in the most humane and civilized manner possible, commensurate with security. Sincerely yours, (signed by the governor)."

A charged silence is broken by the scornful inmate. "The law, the law! As though that can't be changed. My God, isn't it worth changing here—or at least thinking or talking about changing it?"

The doomed man seethes with indignation at what he deems to be the most despicable sort of betrayal, as though some abstract, noble, absolute, transcendental—yet palpable—truth had been desecrated.

The chaplain is keenly aware of what the inmate is driving at and tries vainly to attenuate a wave of disillusionment beginning to engulf his own psyche. "All three say essentially the same thing," he ruminates to himself. "The same prolix niceties—beating around the bush, dodging the issue, and evasive dread of controversy, no matter how lofty, sensible or beneficial the aim."

The last vestige of hope disappears from the convict's eyes as he sits down on the cot. He is calmer now; he realizes that at this late hour there is nothing that the chaplain or anybody else can do. But the doomed man at least relishes the satisfaction of having sensed the chaplain's unspoken approval of and sympathy for his futile desire to donate organs.

In this more tranquil frame of mind the inmate begins to steel himself to face the empty fate ordained for him as well as for many others before (and probably after) him: to leave the "most humane and civilized maintenance commensurate with security" in order to suffer a grotesque, agonizing, and surely *not* most civilized manner of dying in a way having little or no meaning.

Neither did the paradox escape the chaplain's notice.

A somber voice abruptly diverts their attention: "We're ready now!"

The guard stands in the cell's open doorway. It is exactly 11:45 P.M. Only the apprehension of imminent doom is now discernible on the convict's face.

Louisiana's execution chamber. 13 July, 00:15 A.M.

What really happened at this instant? A great deal more than the commissioner, the administrator, the governor, the guards, and the spectators—and perhaps even you, the reader—might think or would care to admit.

It is easy to overlook the fact that the times indicated at the beginning of the narrative of events in all the other states are simultaneous with the time of pronouncement of death for the execution described. So, here's what *really* happened:

A twenty-eight-year-old healthy young man died, partially immolated.

An abstraction called justice was served.

A thirty-nine-year-old wife and mother was condemned to death by renal failure.

An eighteen-year-old youth was condemned to death by renal failure.

A forty-one-year-old father was condemned to death by liver failure.

A thirty-two-year-old wife was condemned to death by heart failure.

A fifty-four-year-old father was condemned to death by lung failure.

A nineteen-year-old youth was condemned to death by lung failure.

Why did all the others die when the criminal was ceremoniously sacrificed on the altar of justice? In the first place, his organs could have been used specifically to save every one of the above patients almost simultaneously; there was plenty of time for carrying out tissue matches and other necessary laboratory studies. If the inmate's organs were to be used in other patients elsewhere, the resultant shortening of the ominous national waiting list would definitely improve prospects for the hypothetical patients depicted and probably rescue them indirectly. No matter how the situation is viewed, it is beyond doubt that the criminal's intention embodied priceless benefits, and that society's blind contempt for him and his autonomy assured conveniently invisible human tragedy of incalculable magnitude.

That's what really happened at fifteen minutes after midnight on 13 July. But, as the executed convict bitterly complained just a half hour earlier, who cares?

It should be pointed out that the three letters read by the chaplain are real, almost word for word. They were received from the quoted authorities in one of our states by an inmate now facing electrocution in that state.

Those authorities certainly don't care.

3

Rebirth of an Idea

Let's turn the clock back even farther, to a crisp and sunny October day in 1958. A light blue, two-door, six-cylinder '56 Ford occasionally exceeds the speed limit south on I-75 toward Columbus, Ohio, with a buoyant thirty-year-old doctor at the wheel. It is his day off from duties as a second-year resident in the Pathology Department of the University of Michigan Medical Center. His buoyancy reflects the zeal of commitment to what he has perceived as a righteous crusade—a self-imposed mission involving diverse academic disciplines and directly or indirectly relevant to all strata of society. In pursuing it he will challenge profound philosophical viewpoints and clash head-on with enduring and powerful taboos.

Unknown to him at the time, his mission actually had begun several months before, at one of those departmental teaching sessions in the autopsy room where once a week the residents were obligated to summarize cases and display gross changes of disease in pieces of organs. During one of these sometimes humdrum exercises there cropped up a moot historical question relating to autopsies, and nobody could answer it. The chief of the department was baffled as well and suggested that the topic would make a good assignment for one of the trainees. Without uttering a word, one of them did decide to take up the challenge, primarily to satisfy his own curiosity. I was that curious doctor. Unfortunately there wasn't a single book dealing with the topic exclusively and comprehensively in our excellent medical library (I couldn't have known, of course, that a couple of good books on the history of dissection were in the process of being published). I therefore had to gather bits of information from various books and journals.

My having studied German paid off when I found plenty of material in often obscure periodicals in that formerly dominant scientific language. One article in particular burned itself indelibly into my memory.[1]* It was a long article replete with detailed interpretation of historical evidence, and it marked a turning point in my career. In time I became convinced that its impact shackled me with the responsibility to promulgate a profound idea which, whether I liked it or not, would somehow and sometime be a major, if not the predominant, goal of my professional life.

With as much detail as is historically justifiable, the author describes how the Ptolemies (kings) of ancient Alexandria decreed that condemned criminals were to be executed by submitting to experimentation in anatomical laboratories. Documented proof from that period has not survived. But it seems that word of the practice reached ancient Rome, where about 400 years after the Alexandrian experience it was recorded (and harshly criticized) by at least two famous historians, Celsus and Tertullian. Many vital details were missing, to be sure; but for me the spark had been lit.

My brief dissertation on the history of the autopsy was well re-

---

*All superscript numbers identify specific references and sources listed at the end of this volume.

ceived by the staff and fellow residents. Shortly thereafter I expanded it into a monograph published in 1959. But my thoughts always returned to and concentrated on those Hellenistic Greek scientists in Alexandria and on what they might have learned during those extraordinary executions. I couldn't help but reflect on the enduring nature of a concept that was well over 2,200 years old. There we were, in 1958, in a country and a world in which condemned criminals were still being executed, at a time when medical research was still a laudable and indispensable activity.

Possibilities churned in my youthful and impractically idealistic mind. How simple a solution to so many perplexing problems. "Surely," I mused, "those civilized and enlightened Greeks must have used some sort of anesthesia on the condemned. Drunken stupor or even alcoholic coma would do it."

At any rate, in the late fifties superb anesthesia was available. That eliminated a major hurdle. Also, it would have to be entirely voluntary on the part of the convicts, which is only fair and decent. Thus, respect for the condemned's personal autonomy eliminated another potential problem for my planned crusade. Therefore, I concluded that our death penalty laws can be so worded as to grant condemned criminals a choice between conventional methods of execution and irreversible surgical depth anesthesia for the purpose of medical experimentation; and that anesthesia would be induced (just as it is routinely in hospitals every day) at the exact instant set for execution by judicial order.

If the subject's live body were to survive the experiment, then a nonphysician technologist or an authorized lay executioner would cause ultimate death with an overdose of anesthetic agent. A neat and very simple concept—and quite different from euthanasia, because it involves more than merciful killing, and a doctor does it.

But I was soon to experience for the first time in my life the enormous force of social, political, and historical inertia which makes it almost impossible to implement seemingly radical change, to bridge the wide gap between rational theory and actual practice.

Despite my ebullient enthusiasm I realized that the possibility of actual change was very remote. The first step would have to be a public explanation of the idea, which I mistakenly assumed to be easy to do and welcome. I was wrong on both counts. Nevertheless, one essential item was still needed to validate the concept and its presentation. I had not yet sampled the opinions of those on death row, to offer evidence that some condemned criminals—indeed just *one*—supported the idea and would like to have the privilege of choice. That called for a visit to death row, to the Ohio Penitentiary since it was the nearest. By mid-afternoon I was making my way through the unfamiliar streets of Columbus.

To one who had never before even seen a large prison, the high, thick, and imposing stone walls of the old edifice were understandably intimidating. With poorly concealed trepidation I proceeded directly to the warden's office.

Only years later, after many formal rebuffs in similar situations, did I realize how naively brazen and audacious I was to barge in on a busy warden as a complete stranger, unannounced, and without prior arrangement. And how lucky I was to have stumbled upon a husky, stern archetype who, contrary to his foreboding demeanor, was interested, honest, and fair enough to patiently weather my deluge of words.

He hardly moved, and uttered nothing after the initial terse greeting. Misinterpreting his unemotional silence as a sure sign of irked disapproval, I hurried to blurt out embellishing details of what I had in mind before getting the expected boot out the door. To my astonishment (and relief) only more silence followed. Then with ineffable joy I watched him call in a lieutenant guard to inquire as to who among the seven convicts then on Ohio's death row might be able to handle such an interview.

Two names were mentioned, and I was instructed to follow the lieutenant as the warden turned to continue working on official papers. It seemed almost incredible that without mincing words, in fact with hardly any conversation, and without any kind of paperwork or formal bureaucratic delay, I was about to experience the key event in the evolution of my mission, the cornerstone of its early development.

Now, years later, I marvel at my sheer blind luck for having encountered Warden Ralph Alvis, one of the very few individuals in any position of authority in any field comprising what is known as "the establishment," who calmly and objectively allowed me to pursue my quest without manifesting a trace of the selfish and Machiavellian hypocrisy that fuels much of civilized society.

My heart began racing as I followed the lieutenant out the rear exit of the warden's office into a large and airy block of cells. At its other end was a metal door through which we entered a long, narrow, windowless corridor. Walking through that passageway was reminiscent of the so-called last mile. Another heavy metal door opened on a tiny cubicle about five feet square and completely enclosed in heavy steel plates. It would have scared any claustrophobic to death!

A couple of light taps form the lieutenant's night stick opened a second door leading out of the cubicle into a much smaller block of cells. Through subdued lighting I could make out a row of small cells along one wall, each of which opened onto a barred corridor made relatively impenetrable by a covering screen of finely meshed but heavy steel wire.

The lieutenant pulled up a chair and stood beside me, motioning for me to sit down. Several cells were empty. The unit's guard entered the corridor, opened the barred gate of one cell, and followed a young, well-built white man to a stool in the corridor directly in front of me.

I was quite apprehensive and suddenly unsure of myself. What heretofore had been safe and comfortable philosophy had now become untested, down-to-earth reality for a neophyte. There I was in the totally alien environment of death row, ready to start talking to a stranger about his excruciating extinction in the electric chair. What was I to say? How to start? This is something I wasn't taught in medical school.

The convict sat quietly and looked me squarely in the eye without emotion, but wondering, I'm sure, what this was all about. I learned later that the twenty-six-year-old inmate had been convicted of murder. The time had come to say something, however inept it might be. A quick search of my memory for a suitable euphemism for execution was fruitless. "You know why you're here," I stammered in a low, almost inaudible voice. No reaction. Definitely a bad start. After only momentary hesitation I continued with a firmer tone: "My being here can't help you, but you can be of great help to me."

That did it. Curiosity lit up in his eyes. With restored confidence I calmly explained why I was there, and he listened silently and with obvious interest for about five minutes. I paused. He looked up at the lieutenant and said, "You know, Lieutenant, maybe they could learn something from my body that might help my little daughter in the future." Turning back to me he averred emphatically that he would choose anesthesia and experimentation if allowed to do so.

I was elated and requested that the inmate put his opinion in writing. He agreed, and about a week later I received that most welcome letter (see figure 1). Misspellings and grammatical errors cannot diminish its eloquence and lofty spirit. At last I knew beyond doubt that the proposal was practical and that the cogent proof was now in my hand. The crusade was unstoppable.

Savoring this initial success, I got up and carried my chair along the screened barrier to face a second inmate seated in the corridor. He was a good looking twenty-year-old black man, the son of a minister, who had murdered a policeman. This inmate was more reserved, aloof, and even somewhat reticent during my presentation. When asked for an opinion, he hesitated ambivalently, saying that he would prefer to talk it over with his wife. But when pressed for an immediate, off-the-cuff decision, he stated a preference for my proposed alternative. In his follow-up letter to me he iterated his wish to postpone a final answer until after having conferred with his wife. I never heard from him again. But the first man's letter was all that I needed.

The return trip to Ann Arbor was one of those rare, exquisitely delightful and all too short episodes that punctuate everyone's lifetime. I immediately set to work composing a short essay outlining the proposal and suggesting how best to implement it. At the outset I stressed my absolute neutrality on the concept of capital punishment itself. I insisted only that there is a far more rational, humane, compassionate, and beneficial way to carry it out.

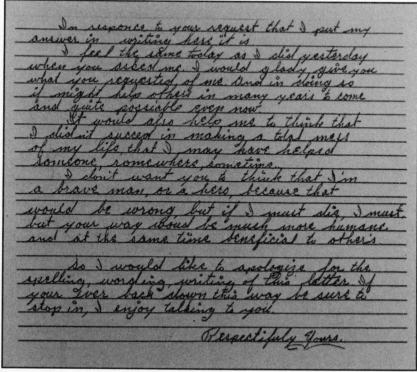

Figure 1. Letter from condemned man in Ohio (October 1958)

Ideally, then, every human being condemned to unavoidable death for any conventional reason—judicial, political, or religious—whether justly or not, anywhere in the world should be allowed this choice: to be executed by the method prescribed by law in the political jurisdiction concerned, or to undergo strictly controlled surgical depth general anesthesia (as used routinely in hospitals every day and therefore safe for the harvesting of all usable body parts) induced precisely at the moment stipulated by law or by the court, and from which there would be no awakening, for the purpose of medical experimentation otherwise impossible to do on living humans.

It need hardly be said that the subject's consent must be firm, unwavering, and based on free access to unlimited medical, legal, and clerical consultation. The choice would not be offered to anyone who manifests ambivalence or uncertainty. Those who decide on anesthesia and experiments would be free to change their minds; but revocation must be limited, say to within one week of the scheduled date of execution (after which the initial assent must stand), in order to avoid the waste of time, effort, and money in preparing for the planned experiments.

This extraordinary opportunity for medical research calls for the utmost concern over what will be done, how it will be done, and who will do it. The "what" is easiest to answer. In every case there must be either an experiment that promises immediate relief of a pressing current need of the largest segment of humanity, or one designed primarily for basic research of no immediate practical importance but aimed solely at expanding our knowledge about what humans really are and what makes us "tick." After all, even "impractical" basic research can have enormous and unforeseen future value. Cardiac catheterization, which opened up the whole field of heart surgery, is an excellent example.

Furthermore, what better circumstances could exist for studying and at least trying to unravel the mechanisms of a criminal mind—a *capitally* criminal mind? We won't get the answers by studying animals; their brains are different. Neither are the answers to be found in brains taken at autopsy. I can state categorically and without fear of contradiction that the only hope for such understanding lies in the study of *all* parts of the intact, *living* brain. That alone is reason enough to take the proposal seriously.

But other body systems also require intensive and deeply probing investigation. Because the demand for experiments would certainly exceed the opportunities offered, great care would have to be taken in selecting those worthy of being performed. Again, ideally, that should be under the aegis of some kind of international panel, perhaps within the structure of the United Nations. It would be responsible for choosing the most promising protocol submitted by research teams throughout the world and matching them with suitable pending executions according to specific criteria—perhaps geographic only.

As far as the "how" is concerned, it seems reasonable to assume that some sort of clinic or laboratory can be set up and equipped to accommodate any type of experiment. Demands for special equipment or personnel could be satisfied by the team chosen to do the research. Such a facility probably should be situated somewhere in the prison, and what better place than in or adjacent to the prison hospital or clinic? If security and an additional possibility of escape are overly worrisome, then the condemned subject could be rendered unconscious in the ordinary execution chamber and kept under anesthesia while transferred to the research facility where the experiment could be completed without the subject ever having regained consciousness.

From personal experience I know that corrections officials oppose these suggestions and oppose granting the condemned such a choice. They seem to be satisfied with the current system of executions with which they are intimately familiar. Their attitude belies the leaden inertia of self-satisfied conservatism, no matter how important the potential change. It is the attitude of most antagonists who, safely insulated from the reality of death row, from life threatening diseases, and from impending death, have the luxury of nonchalantly indulging their thinly veneered hypocrisy with regard to my proposal.

And finally, the "who," the investigators themselves. It would be a unique privilege in the most emphatic sense to be able to experiment on a doomed human being. Therefore, some kind of effort must be made, no matter how intensive or how feeble, and no matter how qualified or incompetent the investigator, to extract *something* of value—no matter how inconsequential—from the execution of every individual who chooses to submit to experimentation.

In an ideal scenario that responsibility would fall to a medical doctor of proven competence in research, of undeniable compassion and dedication, and of impeccable character. They are rare. And like the corrections authorities, they and most of their colleagues, especially those who speak for the profession as a whole, also are antagonists and would refrain from participation—not only because of the same petrified conservatism for which the healing profession is well known, but also because of misguided loyalty to what is now an essentially irrelevant Hippocratic Oath.

Well, then, how about the other kinds of doctors, those ivory-tower Ph.D.s? Surely they're also doing terrific research, and much of it very basic. They could implement the proposal just as well, if not better. I have in mind the memory of our universally liked and respected professor of neuroanatomy at medical school. Here was a Ph.D. who spent countless early morning hours operating on the brains and nervous systems of animals with superb skill and excellent results; who could operate circles around any neurosurgeon on the university staff; and who was always relied on to come up with the correct diagnosis in baffling cases. It staggers me to imagine what that kind of skill and dedication could have accomplished on doomed humans. But without much doubt such Ph.D.s would likewise shy away from mere endorsement, let alone actively taking part—again, on the basis of "ethics," aesthetics, religion, philosophy, or some other visceral emotion or man-made abstraction.

The answer may be to train individuals as special technologists capable of performing the most demanding experiments devised by themselves or by others who refuse to participate actively. Candidates for such training would have to possess the requisite personality in addition to demonstrated mental and physical dexterity. The program could be organized and managed by some governmental agency or perhaps by a respected private organization. In this regard highly motivated lay individuals could take part either as auxiliary support or as chief investigators if everyone else refuses to become involved. The continued reticence now manifested by medical professionals eventually could cost them control of what may become, and should be, a medical specialty.

The stage might already be set for that trend to develop. For example, at least one state legislature is considering a bill that would authorize trained technicians to remove organs for transplantation from clinically brain-dead donors. It only stands to reason that the same approach can be taken with regard to the removal of organs from anesthetized condemned criminals if doctors persist in conjuring up indefensible reasons to abstain and thereby witness the further erosion of their rightful prerogatives. They have not yet learned that, ultimately, unjustified inaction in the face of increasing demand for action eventually leads to the loss of the mandate to act; and that others will assume that mandate.

Finally, somebody invariably raises the specter of the infamous Nazi medical crimes of World War II. That haunting aberration is unfairly compared and even equated with my proposal. There couldn't be a greater difference!

First of all, the Nazis never bothered about consent, informed or not. It wasn't a privilege even to be considered, let alone granted.

Second, anesthesia was rarely if ever used; and when used, it was generally not for the victim's benefit.

Third, many, if not most, of the "experiments" were for rather frivolous aims which could have been achieved faster, easier, and just as accurately in more acceptable ways.

Fourth, most of the "researchers" were given the chance to indulge their often macabre, pseudoscientific whims more as a reward for fanatical loyalty to the regime than as acknowledgment of their scientific acumen.

Fifth, and *most important*, from a legal standpoint the comparison is outrageously absurd. The Nazis condemned people on the basis of highly prejudicial statutes, not at all compatible with international standards, aimed at enforcing strictly arbitrary racial, social, political, and biological dogma. They were enacted by an impotent puppet "legislature" in a totalitarian state at the mercy of a brutal and fanatical autocrat. And the resultant experiments were *wartime* atrocities beyond any hope of civilized control.

On the other hand, peacetime condemnations in the United States are imposed under the most complete, enduring, and modern democratic system of jurisprudence; are fostered by laws compatible with international standards; and guarantee the right of redress and numerous appeals.

To insist on such a comparison denotes an appalling lack of common sense—to say the *very* least.

I realized that the essay I was preparing reeked with sophomoric idealism and was highly impractical. I knew that there was no chance of getting the concept translated into practice, no matter how "prudent" or piecemeal my approach. Indeed, I was soon to learn that it was equally futile to try bringing it up merely for discussion. Since the effect was likely to be the same no matter what I did—namely, complete disinterest or active shunning on the part of those who would listen—I concluded that there was nothing to lose by aiming for the highest theoretical standard of which such a neglected concept is worthy, toward the pure idealism of naivete, "shooting for the moon," so to speak. I decided not to compromise even its most "impractical" implications in the short essay, which I composed in late October of 1958.

After much thought I settled on the title "Capital Punishment or Capital Gain." Its conciseness coupled with the implication of profit or progress and of short- and long-term benefits seemed to more than make up for what might be taken to be a somewhat flippant play on words. To my dismay the article was rejected by editors of several medical journals and popular magazines.

Determined that the idea would at least get an open hearing, I contacted the chairman of the Criminology Section scheduled to participate in the December 1958 annual meeting of the American Association for the Advancement of Science in Washington, D.C. I expected a refusal of my request to include my paper at their session, because the agenda had been set long in advance and the meeting was only two months away. The immediate acceptance took me aback. Only afterwards did I fully grasp why my paper was sandwiched in. It seems that the chairman was an ardent opponent of capital punishment and evidently surmised that the emotionalism engendered would so rekindle memories of the Nazi atrocities as to reinforce and extend sentiment against the death penalty.

My presentation did create quite a stir, in both the listening audience and the press. It received prominent coverage in local evening and weekend newspapers, and was dissemiated nationally through the wire services. However, no significant or serious debate resulted, and no official action or interest was evident. Newspapers reported a few negative medical responses. The only public endorsement reported in the press came from a spokesman for an animal rights group who, with unarguable rationality and logic, could see nothing wrong with a proposal concerning indebted humans who can think and speak, and are free to decide on a strictly human issue.

A definitely positive result of the presentation was an offer to have the essay published in a legitimate journal. The condensed version appeared as a very short article in the June 1959 issue of the *Journal of Criminal Law, Criminology, and Police Science*. From my previous search for source material in libraries and archives, I know that that article is the first documentation in history of the concept for a peacetime society.

Another positive result was the sincere interest shown by a member of that Washington, D.C., audience. He was a professor of sociology from a midwestern state who volunteered to help me sample the opinions of noncondemned prisoners in his state's penitentiary. Because of his previous field research in penology there, he was granted permission in early 1959 to enlist the participation of any willing inmate. He then prepared a concise summary based on my paper and entitled it "Death by the Needle." It was published in the prison newsletter and later reproduced as an introduction to a questionnaire I had prepared and mailed to his office.

It proved difficult to persuade inmates to take part, for several reasons. First, because of the disagreeable nature of the death penalty itself. Second, most of the prisoners opposed the penalty. And finally, such a study seemed to be irrelevant in a state on the verge of abolishing the penalty at the time.

Eventually 104 inmates acceded to the professor's request. Before passing out the questionnaires, he and his staff assistants slowly read the questions aloud and explained in detail the meaning of each. Two weeks later I received the good news that 89 of the participants (85 percent) endorsed the proposal, and that the professor planned to have the results published.

The outcome is even more significant in retrospect because the inmates' opinions dealt with my original (and apparently still much too "radical") intention of conducting medical experimentation only. This was a time when organ transplantation was merely theoretical and not at all the practical imperative it is today. That, in all likelihood, is why the professor encountered among his own colleagues the same antagonism I met in the ranks of medicine. No sociological journal would accept our jointly authored paper, and the survey remained unpublished.

Zealous activism on this issue had unexpected but certainly understandable repercussions on my professional career from the start, even before my presentation at the Criminology Section seminar. This is understandable considering that the negative responses from medical journals had made me aware for the first time of the well-disguised myth that they and the academic institutions they represent are bastions of a free exchange of ideas. They are—but only of those ideas that don't "rock the boat," that refrain from challenging hallowed taboos. Mine did both.

So, I was not caught by surprise when a staff professor and friend approached me, evidently charged with the odious task of giving me a rare ultimatum: either I drop the controversial death penalty campaign or leave the residency program at the university. The decision was easy, not the least important reason being my desire to learn how pathology is taught and practiced in the real world of a busy city general hospital. I resigned.

Fortunately (for me) there was a doctor shortage at the time, and it was not difficult to secure another position. Without rancor or regret I left my friends in the exalted but philosophically stultified milieu of Academe to enter a less prestigious realm which, I was delighted to find, proved to be professionally satisfying and offered absolutely no obstacles to my plans.*

During the following year I corresponded with the chairman of a special committee formed to consider possible revision of Ohio's

---

*I became a third-year resident in pathology at Pontiac (Michigan) General Hospital.

death penalty law. Its recommendations were ready for legislative debate by April 1960, and at my request I was invited to testify before a joint judiciary committee meeting in Columbus. I brought along packets containing copies of my first essay, my newly published monograph, and supportive letters from several researchers as well as from two theologians (one Catholic, one Protestant).

The packets were handed out to the committee members, who were seated around a large rectangular conference table. Their facial expressions ranged from blank to skeptical as I began speaking. But that didn't bother me much: my total consciousness and mental energy were immersed in the essence of the matter that brought me there, and I was completely oblivious of all else. Near the end of my impassioned plea, which lasted about twenty minutes, I was delighted to sense success from the many cordial smiles of apparent agreement.

A front-page report in the local newspaper the next day quoted one of the legislators as having remarked that he at first thought I was a crackpot but changed his mind as he listened. Another committee member admitted being so impressed that he was considering the introduction of an enabling bill. But such a move would have been ill-timed, because there was a rising tide of sentiment against capital punishment, which would eventually have invalidated the contemplated legislation. The changing mood compelled me to stop all activity; otherwise I might have been wrongly accused of striving to foster use of the death penalty itself.

My monograph, published at my own expense, was entitled *Medical Research and the Death Penalty*. Its dialogue format seemed to offer the best means of summarizing pro and con arguments. Most reviews were favorable, including one published in the *Journal of the American Medical Association* (*JAMA*), which was remarkable in view of its editors' rejection of my original essay. Another perceptive reviewer came close to the truth by concluding that the idea's complete rationality is perhaps its greatest weakness. But that is turning things around. What the reviewer should have said is that the idea's complete rationality merely evokes a weakness already inherent in those who oppose it.

In the course of that published dialogue, I anticipated the introduction of lethal drug injection by suggesting that the condemned be allowed to choose anesthesia alone, without experimentation—a suggestion which met with the approval of JAMA's book reviewer. But that was contrary to AMA's attitude years later when lethal injection was being considered by the Oklahoma legislature.

My campaign ground to a halt as the death penalty fell into disuse over the next decade and a half. Perhaps merely out of habit I occasionally would stop at nearby prisons when traveling for various unrelated reasons, and request permission to speak with a few men still languishing on inactive death rows. But the good luck in Columbus was never repeated.

The fact that death rows existed throughout the moratorium was a good sign that a prediction made in my 1960 monograph was on target: the unstoppable pendulum of history would bring with its next swing a resumption of executions. There was no doubt in my mind that the total and permanent abolition of capital punishment is a delusion of wishful sentimentality trying vainly to insulate itself from the harsh realities of human nature. And I was determined to "pull out all stops" when that swing back gathered momentum.

It happened in the mid-1970s as a result of two factors. The first was the sensational Gary Gilmore case in Utah. The plight of that brutal but glib murderer had become the rallying point for vociferous opponents of capital punishment and had fanned passionate interest here and abroad.

The sensationalism was enhanced by the unusual prospect of Gilmore's execution by firing squad. His situation seemed to offer a good opportunity for me to start again, especially because Utah at that time already offered the condemned a choice in the method of execution (between hanging and firing squad). I hoped to persuade authorities to extend the choice to include my suggestion, but first I had to know how Gilmore might respond. My hopes faded when in a telephone conversation with Gilmore's attorney I was told that the condemned criminal wanted a "messy" death and wouldn't dream of choosing to die anesthetized. Shortly thereafter four bullets shattered his heart—and started the pendulum's swing back.

The second crucial development was the rapid growth of organ transplantation. Here at last was an invincible argument for the granting of a choice to permit the procurement of precious vital organs in the best possible condition in order to save the lives of several dying patients.

Theoretically (and probably in practice, too), a single healthy condemned inmate could be the salvation of at least six doomed adults by offering two biologically robust kidneys, two "clean" lungs, a heart, and a liver; and, in addition, save two more by donating a fresh pancreas and small intestines. That adds up to a total of eight lives, but the precious transfer of life and death need not end there. If the condemned's liver were surgically divided, then two dying infants could also be saved, raising to nine the number of lives salvaged by one inmate. And a bone marrow transplant could save a tenth patient.

Surgeons in Chicago have pioneered the transplantation of part of a parent's liver into his or her doomed baby. The operation was hailed as a great "breakthrough" by the news media, but it could have been done long before with the livers of willing condemned men. The technique was already developed; and there can be no doubt that the reluctance of surgeons to use such donations from men executed during the last several years has resulted in the tragic and unnecessary death of many infants; worse yet, it has forced (and will continue to force) parents to make the unnecessary biological sacrifice of part of a vital organ.

By no stretch of the imagination could there be greater or more meaningful retribution in connection with capital punishment. From this point on I openly deemed opposition to my proposal from legislative authorities and doctors to be a sign of their pathetic mental or spiritual infirmity.

The next significant event for me took place a year and a half later, in 1979, at which time an Alabama inmate named John Evans was scheduled to die in the electric chair. Although time was short, I sent him a letter together with explanatory material, and requested a personal interview. There was no reply. However, at the same time, it occurred to me that I had never received the opinions of those directly affected by the results of the condemned man's crimes, the family members of the victims. By telephone I arranged to meet one victim's close relative outside of the prison on the morning of the day set for execution. It turned out to be a poor arrangement. I failed to locate the individual in the huge crowd milling about the spacious grounds that morning. But my trip to Atmore Prison was not in vain.

While scanning the throng, I spotted a pensive man walking slowly and apparently aimlessly in my direction. I took the liberty of greeting him, and soon we were discussing what was on everybody's mind that day. My spirits picked up when I learned that he was a prominent figure in the American Civil Liberties Union (ACLU), an organization about which I knew little at the time, but which I assumed would be glad to endorse my campaign. My assumption was wrong, very wrong.

It astounded me that a supposedly intelligent and rational man could come out with such irrelevant and even nonsensical "arguments" against my position. He doggedly insisted that it was better to let Evans be electrocuted than to let him choose to be anesthetized. It has always been difficult for me to abide irrational discourse with someone expected and reputed to know better—especially if it is *feigned and deceitful* merely to affect public opinion. And I reacted accordingly.

The rising volume of our increasingly angry voices drew the attention of a few news reporters casually conversing a short distance away. Hoping for something newsworthy, they hastened over. As a dozen or so crowded around us, my adversary suddenly became apprehensive and stopped talking. I sensed his impending retreat and quickly tried to explain to the reporters, who by then were ready with pad and pencil, exactly what was going on and what was being said. In the meantime the ACLU poltroon had slunk (literally) out of the group, with head bowed and turned away as though dreading identification, while I shouted after him: "Come back you coward! Come back and say what you just said to me!" Of course I knew he wouldn't dare. He couldn't risk having such nonsense from a highly placed official of the ACLU disseminated to the press for all to read. So, like a chastised dog with a shamefully dangling tail he disappeared into the sanctuary of the crowd.

At that moment I understood clearly that the ACLU is a self-righteous organization devoted to the pursuit of an arbitrarily contrived concept of human rights. Years later this conclusion was reinforced independently by letters I received from several condemned men. They also are now aware of the ACLU's crafty bias.

Late in the afternoon it was announced tht Evans had been granted a reprieve, and the crowd quickly dispersed. I returned home rather disappointed at the lack of any kind of positive outcome from my standpoint. I was unaware that during the next few years the same condemned man had started his own campaign to donate organs, perhaps motivated by the material I had sent him in 1979. But Evans's pleas and lucid arguments were ignored, and he was electrocuted in 1983.

As the number of sporadic executions grew, my one-man campaign shifted into high gear. Over the previous several years I had prepared four articles, which no American medical journal would accept. Fortunately Judge Amnon Carmi, the editor of *Medicine and Law*, an international journal based in Israel, was less intimidated by potential controversy and saw fit to give my views a fair hearing.

The first of this series of papers denounced organized medicine's unjustifiable opposition to lethal injection as a method of execution, even as a choice among more gruesome alternative methods. It also criticized the profession's official position prohibiting doctors from performing the injections on the basis of outmoded ethical precepts, emotional revulsion, philosophical or religious tenets, and threat of professional censure.[2]

The next paper aimed to undermine the profession's antipathy toward the use of anesthesia during executions for the purpose of experimentation or organ procurement by presenting the results of my own public opinion poll conducted in Long Beach, California, in 1984.[3] It is the only study of its kind, patterned after the ill-fated questionnaire project on 1959 but expanded to include the possibility of organ donation. The majority of five social classes polled endorsed what the medical profession officially shies away from. The participants included both condemned and noncondemned convicts, college students, medical personnel, and ordinary citizens.

The third article advocated and offered a working model for a new bioethical code dealing specifically with the proposed practices —a code that currently does not exist, and never existed (see the Appendix).[4] All other prior codes dodged the topic completely—that includes the highly regarded and frequently cited Nuremberg code, which is supposed to have solved a problem it didn't even address!

The final paper in the series aimed for the future. It advocated extension of the concept to include extraction of medical benefit from the extraordinary possibilities made accessible when and if voluntary euthanasia is officially sanctioned everywhere (as it is now in the Netherlands) and eventually legitimated (as it surely will be some day).[5]

In the meantime I learned another hard lesson: erudite articles ceremoniously buried in genteel academic journals did little or nothing (mostly the latter) for the advancement of my campaign. Therefore, I decided that the incubation period had gone on far too long. The time had come to transform my almost ludicrous one-man campaign into more of the mass movement needed to nudge and guide a smugly complacent society toward implementation of a more rational mechanism for the excretion of that small portion of humanity that society wrongly deems to be waste material.

But, how to go about it, and whom to enlist? Corrections and prison officials were resistant. Medical authorities were appalled. Theologians were somewhat aloof and split. And legislators were mute or evasive.

It became apparent that the pressure had to well up from the cellar of society: from a lone doctor at the bottom rung of his calling, without authority, influence, or organizational support (and ultimately even without a job) combined with the absolute lowest of the low, the condemned criminals themselves. Nevertheless, in this unlikely union I sensed a unique source of power, and concentrated on tapping it to the limits of my meager resources. I would have to contact as many death row inmates as possible in order to put together a chorus of voices—the voices that really count—which couldn't help but be heard and perhaps even heeded.

In 1984, I began collecting from newspaper accounts the names of condemned men and women, in various states, whose latest appeals had been rejected by the U.S. Supreme Court; and I sent them a letter of inquiry with explanatory material enclosed. At first I mistakenly assumed that every reported rejection concerned a final appeal and that execution was imminent in every case. I soon learned from their replies that the lengthy judicial process can entail up to nine separate appeals.

Of the many male inmates contacted, about one out of every six or seven answered. Only one of five women responded; hers was a short, noncommittal, indeed unintelligible comment.

A few of the men gave only qualified approval of my proposal, but the majority endorsed it unconditionally—some with just a sentence or two, and others with several pages of eloquent praise. One inmate, sentenced to be electrocuted, wanted to make some sort of "deal" before giving me his support, which surely is not altruistic. I rejected that idea immediately, before any details could be spelled out. Another convict who faced electrocution sent me a very sarcastic, vulgar letter of rejection containing many expletives—it arrived over a year after I had written to him. These few, starkly negative responses were a valuable reminder that all inmates on death row are not "nice guys" and that malice still reigns there.

Nevertheless, the power in the words of the letters of endorsement proved that my hunch was on the right track. A combination of growing pressure from the condemned on the inside with similar pressure from me on the outside was beginning to bear fruit. A few state legislators started to pay attention, and a couple even began to act. The news media also got interested again, albeit sporadically.

But by far the most important result was the evolution of a tiny but real movement now energized by more than myself. Several equally dedicated residents of death row are now working with me to persuade the public and its lawmakers to offer the condemned, when their time comes, the opportunity to suffer the supreme penalty in a way that befits civilized society.

4

Sentenced to What Kind of Death?

The method of execution has somehow always fulfilled the aims of torture and revenge—nowadays surreptitiously—and usually in a highly dramatic way. The ancient Hebrews and Assyrians buried the condemned alive. Crucifixion was also popular, until abolished by Constantine in A.D. 325. It was usually performed by breaking the condemned's leg bones, sitting him on a bar fastened to the post of a wooden cross, and pinning his now very flexible legs beneath him with a nail through the feet. The outstretched arms were attached to the crossbar with nails through the hands, and the victim was allowed to suffer there until dead.[6]

During mass executions in the Roman Coliseum many simultaneously crucified criminals were smeared with tar and set ablaze at night to form spectacular human torches.[7] The ancient Greeks used the wheel, later resurrected in sixteenth-century France and Germany.

In this method a heavy bar or hammer was used to break almost every bone in the limbs, hips, and shoulders of a victim who had been laid flat on a horizontal wheel. The flail limbs were braided around the rim. Death resulted either from blows to the chest and head, or from prolonged exposure aloft on the elevated wheel.[8]

Men, and especially women, in pre-Christian Britain and Rome were executed by drowning in ponds and marshes. During these early times beheading by sword was also common and generally reserved for highly respected or aristocratic individuals.[9] This tradition continued into nineteenth-century Europe.

In eighth-century England the Danes executed criminals by throwing them off cliffs. A century or so later the Britons resorted to the ancient practice of stoning people to death. In thirteenth-century England the gibbet appeared and became so popular that gallows were to be seen almost everywhere.[6]

The gibbet was the forerunner of modern hanging. The victim was placed in chains, or in a specially constructed body cage of latticed iron, and hoisted onto a wooden crossbar. He hung there until dead or until some compassionate countryman killed him to end his suffering. It wasn't until the eighteenth century that the "drop" (the counterpart of our modern trapdoor) was introduced. The assumption was (and apparently still is) that breaking the condemned's neck was a more "humane" way to kill. This method is still in use today in the United States.

Criminals were burned alive in wicker baskets as sacrifices to gods in pre-Christian Europe.[6] At the same time burning alive at the stake was common in Britain, a method used for the wholesale slaughter of many thousands of heretics* and apostates during the Middle Ages. The agony of victims was frequently eased by compassionate executioners who would subtly tighten the restraining cord around the neck for a tolerable death by strangulation before flames reached the flesh.[10]

---

*At least one, Dr. Viethes of Hamburg, was sentenced to death in 1521 for the capital crime of ameliorating the pain of a woman in labor (D. T. Atkinson, *Magic, Myth, and Medicine* [Cleveland: World Publishing, 1956], p. 272).

Other novel and gruesome methods were devised by the end of the sixteenth century. In Russia some criminals were dragged to death tied to the tails of horses, while others were strapped to the backs of wild beasts and sent off to die in the forests.[6] In England they were sometimes pressed to death under increasingly heavier weights. Occasionally the victim's friends would add their own body weight to the load to cut short the suffering.[9] In Spain execution often was by garrotting, through the tightening of a steel collar against a backboard until the neck was broken. Whipping to death with intertwined thongs and metal wires was common in medieval Britain and Russia. Boiling to death was used for a short while in England under Henry VIII.[9] And in India the criminal lay on the ground or knelt over a tree stump to have his head squashed under an elephant's foot.[11]

A couple of particularly repugnant methods were used in China. One consisted of placing live criminals in crude coffins and sawing them in half lengthwise from head to crotch.[10] This unspeakably brutal method was used in Spain as late as the nineteenth century, where the victim was sawn while positioned upside down to intensify and prolong the suffering.[8] The Chinese also resorted to the so-called thousand cuts whereby an executioner would slowly and deliberately cut into and cut off parts of the body so skillfully that death occurred only after the thousandth cut.[10] This extraordinary ritual made allowances for gradations of condemnation: executions with less rancor called for the curtailed suffering of only ten or one hundred cuts.

Constant complaints from executioners in medieval England about difficulty in keeping their swords sharp and keeping many restive criminals in place during decapitation led to the development of "beheading machines." The earliest examples appeared in thirteenth-century Europe. The English model, called the Halifax gibbet, made use of an axe blade having its butt end affixed to a heavy wooden block which moved freely between two vertical guide rails of wood.[9] The block was raised by a rope pulled by men or animals, and it dropped suddenly on release of the rope to lop off the head of a criminal lying prone on a bench. As a rule the severed head would sometimes roll on the ground for a considerable distance. This contraption obviously was the forerunner of the infamous guillotine used (indeed overused) during the French Revolution. (More will be said in chapter 10 about that once extremely popular device.)

Without much doubt the most gruesome method in the Western world was drawing and quartering.[6] In the Middle Ages the procedure consisted of having horses drag (or draw) a criminal to a public square. Drawing alone caused so much physical trauma and even occasional death that, in time, a type of sledge was used to carry the criminal behind the horse. At the square the criminal was hanged on a gibbet, later taken down alive, disemboweled, and then decapitated. The headless body was then cut into quarters and all parts were stuffed into a basket for public display.

The most horrendous example took place in France in 1757. A very strong and husky man named Damiens was condemned to death for the attempted assassination of Louis XV. Damiens's request for a quick death was denied. Instead the hand that held the gun was soaked in oil and burned off, and molten sulfer was poured over the stump. Then he was laid out supine in the public square. Six horses were brought in, and the executioner bound one horse to each of Damiens's outstretched arms and two horses to each of his legs. Incredibly the animals strained for almost two hours under whip lashes, but Damiens's limbs stayed intact. Then to make the horses' terrible task easier, the desperate executioner cut into the man's hip and shoulder joints. It worked, as first one, then another leg tore off and then an arm. The last attached arm pulled the trunk a short distance where it lay, still apparently alive according to witnesses who said that the head and arm rose a bit and the lips moved as if trying to speak before falling dead. All the body parts were then burned and the ashes spread over the square.[6]

This was happening at a time when serious debate was beginning to rage over the morality of judicial killing and over the relative merits of how it was done. Humanitarian demands for less torturous methods seemed to be on the verge of satisfaction when thoughts turned in the late nineteenth century to the increasing knowledge and practical application of electricity. At the same time, legislators and penal authorities in the State of New York resolved that shooting and hanging were too gruesome; they opted instead for the "clean" method of electrocution. Their specially built mahogany chair was used for the first time to execute a murderer in August 1890.[11]

The novelty quickly spread to other states, despite official reports of unintentional agonizing results from prolonged electrocution due to equipment failure, misjudgment of body resistance, and bickering among officials about who was to throw the switch. In fact, the hypothetical but credible event described in chapter 1 is mild compared to a real electrocution which went awry in Alabama in 1983, during which three separate attempts were required to kill the criminal. Witnesses reported seeing flickering flames beneath the face mask, and tissues around the electrodes were charred black.

Similar bad experiences with electrocution in the opening decade of the present century prompted authorities in Nevada to turn to the use of hydrogen cyanide as the death-dealing agent, and in 1924 the gas chamber made its debut.[11]

Lethal injection rounds out the brief history of execution methods into the late twentieth century. This technique caused a serene, rapid death from the intravenous injection of three drugs in mixed solution: a fast-acting barbiturate for almost instantaneous unconsciousness, a muscle paralyzer to stop breathing and to avert convulsions, and potassium chloride to stop the heart. It was adopted as the official method by the Oklahoma legislature in 1977, but was first used in Texas in 1982.

From this review one might conclude that methods of execution have become progressively more humane during the present century. However, a valid assessment demands critical analysis of the mechanism involved for each method. Let's start with the first "modern" technique: the electric chair.

Electricity causes biological damage through both heat and electrochemical havoc. Heat denatures (or inactivates) protein by coagulating it, thereby doing away with its biological function through the destruction of enzymes, hormones, and even tissue structure. The electrical current itself nullifies the function of organs and tissues such as the brain, nerves, and heart by overwhelming the fragile bioelectrical basis of their metabolism. The voltage applied is not the critical factor but is, in fact, almost irrelevant as mere electrical "pressure."

The body can tolerate millions of volts without discomfort. High school physics students often delight in making their hair stand on end by taking a high-voltage charge from an electrostatic generator. It is the amperes that do the heating and electrical damage; they comprise the actual current driven by the pressure of volts.

The type of electrical current, too, makes a difference—whether direct (DC) or alternating (AC). The latter is more dangerous and can be lethal even with low voltage and relatively low amperage. The alternating cycle of 60 per second, which is ordinary 110-120 volt house current, can be extremely dangerous and, without producing excessive heating, will invariably stop heart action through standstill or ventricular fibrillation if the body somehow becomes part of the circuit. That often happens accidentally in the home when someone's body is immersed in or in good contact with water, which reduces the ordinarily strong skin resistance and turns the body into an electrical conductor. Therefore, high voltage and amperage used in the electric chair may be awesome and spectacular, but totally unnecessary and unduly torturous.

When sodium cyanide pellets are dropped into acid beneath the seated subject in a gas chamber, extremely lethal hydrogen cyanide (chemical symbol HCN) is produced. As a medical student I saw a demonstration using a rabbit that had been given a solution of sodium cyanide via a stomach tube. Within 35-40 seconds the animal began leaping about in convulsions and dropped dead about 15 seconds later.

Cyanide asphyxiates by choking the cells instead of blocking air intake. The gas, HCN, is rapidly absorbed into the bloodstream through the lungs—much faster than a solution of cyanide is absorbed through the stomach. The red blood cells are relatively immune to HCN, because most of their hemoglobin iron is in a reduced state (Fe I or Fe^{++}) for which the poison has little affinity. But when delivered to all other body cells, the cyanide penetrates the cells' tiny energy-producing centers (called mitochondria) and quickly inactivates the mitochondrial enzymes (cytochrome oxidases) that are necessary if oxygen is to assist in the production of energy. These cytochrome enzymes are highly susceptible to attack because their iron is in the trivalent (Fe II or Fe^{+++}) form. In this way cyanide literally and rapidly chokes all the body's cells to death at the same time.

It doesn't take much HCN to induce death: concentrations of as little as 200-300 parts of cyanide per million parts of air can do it. Actually two mechanisms are involved. One is a direct toxic effect on the central nervous system, which controls breathing. The other is the choking effect already described. Both combine to deprive the heart and brain of oxygen, thereby triggering ultimate cessation of heart function (and perhaps some muscle twitches or even frank convulsion in the agony of death, as in the case of the rabbit).

Oxygen deprivation also is the cause of death in drowning and strangulation or garrotting. Contrary to popular belief, in drowning the lungs do not always fill with water. In fact, in some instances very little water enters the lungs, because when water hits the glottis (the opening between the two vocal cords) a quick reflex shuts it to keep the water out (as it would any material foreign to the trachea). That allows a submerged body to keep a small amount of residual air in the lungs and oxygen in the bloodstream for a short while longer.

In garrotting, the neck is slowly but forcefully broken and the upper spinal cord severely crushed or torn. The damage could extend to higher levels in the medulla* or pons,† either mechanically through stretching or laceration, or physiologically through so-called spinal shock. Centers for the regulation of breathing and heart action are located in that vital area. Their destruction or impairment could result in immediate cessation of breathing and heartbeat and a death perhaps faster than that due to drowning.

Anyone who has witnessed the decapitation of a chicken has a

---

*Medulla oblongata—brain stem.
†Pons—part of the base of the brain.

pretty good idea of how a headless human body might react. The fowl's wild thrashing about, as if in panic, suggests purposeful, if unconscious, action. It is easy to assume that the action is totally unconscious, because it is also assumed (in fact, almost axiomatic) that consciousness resides in the brain, which would no longer be functional after decapitation.

But that which we now take for granted was the subject of intensive debate and research in nineteenth-century Europe: does consciousness persist for any time at all after decollation? The question was important because the number of executions by sword and guillotine was large and increasing during a simultaneous wave of humanitarian concern sweeping the continent.

There were many severed heads to study. From observation of muscular reactions to mechanical and electrical stimuli applied to various parts of the head, including the cut ends of muscles and spinal cord in the neck, one group of investigators concluded that perception of pain persists for a short interval, perhaps as long as fifteen minutes after beheading.[12] But even obvious muscular reaction was considered to be irrelevant as an indicator of functional integrity of the nervous system. This group theorized that it might be kept intact in a detached head by small amounts of slowly moving blood trapped in the network of finer vessels.

But another research team disagreed emphatically.[12] This latter group postulated that consciousness was due to some sort of ethereal life essence that they called "nerve fluid." The flow of that hypothetical "fluid" through nerves toward the brain supposedly produced awareness; and away from the brain, as would be the case with massive drainage of the "fluid" from the nervous tissue transected by the decapitation, would have to result in instantaneous unconsciousness.

The controversy became very heated and so popular that it was made a regular feature in daily newspapers. Such research and argumentation may strike us today as having been unsophisticated, sophomoric, even silly. Nevertheless the investigators involved were dedicated men of integrity and competence. And in comparing the times and resources at hand, was their predicament really much different from the current state of affairs with regard to the enigma of AIDS, for example, which emblazons the pages of our newspapers and magazines? After all, theirs was a much tougher and more basic problem; they tackled something that was probably beyond the scope of science or any human capability.

Like decapitated fowl, the headless human body has also demonstrated apparently purposeful action. In some instances of judicial decapitation the headless body had to be forcefully held to prevent it from springing up.[10] And early in the twentieth century a few sadistic officers in the army of the Shah of Iran would, for their own amusement, bet on how far a standing condemned man could run after having been beheaded by sword. One by one the victims had their heads lopped off as they started to run. Some of them ran for considerable distances.[13] That probably manifested an unconscious reflex action somehow preprogrammed into lower nerve centers, either as a final conscious act of a brain aware of its impending destruction, or simply by virtue of the action having been an ongoing muscular process with—quite suddenly—nothing left to influence it until complete exsanguination cut off the source of energy.

The question of how hanging affects consciousness soon complicated matters. Proponents of hanging as a more humane method objected to the practice of beheading: they maintained that there was no way to disprove the possibility that traces of consciousness exist in severed heads even when the so-called nerve fluid drained from the brain. Furthermore, they argued that the damage caused by the trauma of transection may be accompanied by temporary numbness which, however, might then be dispelled by another powerful stimulus. That could happen, they continued, when the blade of the sword or guillotine strikes violently through the complex nervous structures concentrated in the upper neck, causing perhaps fleeting pain followed immediately by numbness. Then the sudden jarring blow of the severed head hitting a basket or the ground could dispel the numbness and result in the perception of excruciating pain.

This remarkable hypothesis seems to have anticipated the recently discovered fact that the brain produces tiny amounts of its own internal analgesic to ameliorate or block the perception of pain due to trauma somewhere in the body. Those agents, called endorphins, are many times more powerful than morphine, and may be the real counterpart of the previously imaginary "nerve fluid."

Turning from criticism of beheading, the advocates of hanging then extolled the merits of their preferred method. They argued that if the noose is correctly applied to the neck, consciousness would disappear quickly due to the sudden and complete damming of blood in the head, with resultant swelling of the brain and rupture of small blood vessels. As proof they cited the testimony of individuals who had been rescued from the gallows: these people swore that there was no pain before they lost consciousness (which sort of "proof," unfortunately, was not available to proponents of beheading). They could recall only occasional flashes of light and the sound of bells. Irritation of the brain could adequately account for such hallucinations, either mechanically from swelling and hemorrhage, or chemically from the progressive deprivation of oxygen due to stagnant circulation.

In all likelihood the same phenomena account for the "near death" experiences being reported with increasing frequency by persons whose romanticism tends to trivialize the profundity and, by strict definition, the irreversibility of that ultimate mystery.[14] As a youngster I, too, can remember similar flashing and shimmering lights (without the sound of bells) that eerily waxed and waned in my ebbing consciousness during ether anesthesia for surgery. It was not pleasant, to say the least.

In a sense any advantages of hanging would seem to have been compromised when the "drop" was added. That embellishment usually results in the breaking of the neck and the ripping of the spinal cord, thus essentially and much more crudely duplicating the results of decapitation without detaching the head (although there have been cases of hanging in which the head of a thin, poorly muscled person was completely torn off after an unusually long drop through the trapdoor).

Proponents of hanging were then embarrassed at having to face the criticism they originally leveled at beheading. Psychologically it is more seductive to imagine residual consciousness in an attached head than in a severed, sickly pale head bled out in a basket. Certainly the effect of "spinal shock" would be the same for both methods. And whereas it would be reasonable to assume consciousness benumbed by cutting or tearing of the spinal cord, might not the opposite be true? Maybe the very violent trauma to the central nervous system would trigger chaotic electrochemical storms to inundate the last vestiges of consciousness with a kaleidoscope of nightmarish images beyond description. The same may be true in cases of death by any method that deprives the brain of oxygen. We can speculate, but there is no way for anyone to know.

Finally, a word about incineration. Again, we are left to guess at the exact mechanism. Possibly death is due to a combination of causes. Victims of accidental death by fire may experience terrible pain from burns on the exterior of the body; but before heat reaches the well-protected vital internal organs to coagulate protein, death usually ensues from inhalation of smoke and carbon monoxide or other toxic gases.

Does the same explanation apply to those who were burned alive at the stake? There is no way of knowing. In such cases many variables would come into play, such as the local atmospheric and climatic conditions, the degree of openness of the site, and the type of fuel used. It is conceivable that some fuels could produce enough toxic gas to cause a more tolerable death by suffocation (comparable to drowning) before the searing of the flesh is perceived.

It is odd that the states whose legislatures resorted to the use of the gas chamber picked hydrogen cyanide over carbon monoxide (chemical symbol CO). Both gases are very lethal; but CO is less toxic and requires a much higher concentration to kill rapidly (10,000 parts of CO per million parts of air will kill an average adult in five minutes). Instead of poisoning enzymes as HCN does, CO merely blocks the transfer of oxygen to red cells in the circulating blood. Carbon monoxide does this easily because its affinity for attaching to hemoglobin is 250 *times* greater than that of oxygen. Therefore, little or no oxygen is available in CO-saturated blood to get into the cells and mitochondria for energy production. In contrast to HCN, CO deprives cells of oxygen from the outside. Yet for both gases the end result is the death of cells from oxygen deprivation.

But it's a different matter when it comes to the economics of running a gas chamber. Carbon monoxide offers a big saving in cost, ease of handling, safety, and probably even a better "quality" of dying.

In the first place, CO is cheaper and widely available in tanks and canisters of various sizes. This abundance of choice offers wide latitude in deciding on chamber construction and gas administration. In fact, a chamber isn't needed at all. Enough CO mixed with air for a relatively quick death can be administered safely by attaching a small tube from the canister or tank to a small, tight-fitting plastic mask over the nose and mouth—similar to the way oxygen is sometimes administered. But that method of dying probably wouldn't be spectacular enough for some people. Furthermore, the concentration of CO being delivered in that way could be precisely controlled, either in the chamber or by mask, through the manipulation of gauges and valves which are not involved in the use of HCN.

It is general knowledge that many accidental deaths from CO occur while the victim remains calmly asleep, which proves that it can be a very serene and tolerable way to put a criminal to death. However, in the case of a conscious individual, the rapid deprivation of oxygen resulting from a sudden, massive dose of CO could conceivably cause rather violent muscular reactions and outright convulsions. That complication probably could be averted by fine tuning a lower concentration of the gas in a specified period of time. As mentioned above, such a technique is possible with tanked CO but not when cyanide pellets are dropped indiscriminately into a receptacle of acid.

Execution by lethal gas is not a twentieth-century invention. Carbon monoxide was used for that purpose in ancient Greece and Rome. All things considered, in this respect it is clear that society hasn't changed much in over 2,000 years. On the contrary, we seem to have slid backwards by choosing HCN—an inferior agent—over carbon monoxide.

The situation is the same with the electric chair. It was originally devised to ease the anguish of dying. In practice it turned out to combine the terrific jolt of an electrical "sword" with the scorching heat of a red-hot pyre around a wooden stake. The combination unmistakably denotes retrogression, and our society is still on this course.

What about lethal injection? Surely that recent innovation constitutes definite progress. After all, thousands of times every day hospitals patients are calmly put under anesthesia for surgery with initial injections of thiopental* and succinylcholine, the same drugs condemned criminals get when executed. The big difference is, of course, that the patients don't get lethal doses, and they revive to tell how tolerable it was. So, that *must* be progress in the way capital punishment is meted out.

Well, let's take a closer look. Thiopental sodium is a fast-acting barbiturate that produces almost instantaneous short-term unconsciousness after a single dose. It is also used as a "truth serum" administered in small, intermittent, carefully calibrated hypnotic doses while the subject counts backward from 100. A trance-like semiconsciousness is usually reached before the count gets to 90.

Succinylcholine is a muscle paralyzer. For the most part it has replaced an older drug, curare, which South American Indians extracted from jungle plants for centuries for use in hunting as poison on the tips of their blowgun darts. By paralyzing the muscles of the body, succinylcholine counteracts the tendency of thiopental to cause muscle tremors or more violent contractions. That assures a surgeon that the patient's body will remain calm and at complete rest, and an executioner that the condemned's body will not react.

To complete the lethal mixture for execution, society has stipulated the addition of potassium chloride. A high level of potassium in the blood paralyzes the heart muscle. In effect, then, that would correspond to a heart attack for the condemned while in the deep

---

*Thiopental can be obtained only by those who possess both state and federal licenses to procure controlled substances as well as a professional license (e.g., doctors, dentists, pharmacists, etc.).

sleep of barbiturate coma (which certainly cannot be said to be cruel or barbaric).

As was the case with electrocution, lethal injection soon spread to other states in short order and is now fast becoming predominant. As of April 1991, the method of execution in twenty-one states is lethal injection. Six states grant a choice: between lethal injection and the gas chamber in Missouri and North Carolina, hanging in Montana and Washington, or a firing squad in Idaho and Utah. There is little doubt that from an objective standpoint it is the method of choice at present, especially as far as those who observe executions are concerned. But, according to some critics, that may not be true for the condemned.

Like its predecessors, lethal injection as now practiced may be melodrama with the inherent risk of overkill. Critics argue that the combination of drugs raises the possibility of a sometimes prolonged an unintentionally agonizing death. For example, if the doses of thiopental and potassium chloride are not big enough to cause immediate death, the condemned could slowly suffocate because of the succinylcholine's paralysis of muscles used for breathing; and the total paralysis of all muscles would make it impossible for even a conscious subject to make that known. According to a few witnesses, that rare possibility may have already happened during recent executions.

Another drawback of lethal injection is in the name itself—injection. It implies the need for a specially trained and very skillful "executioner." Currently doctors are exempt by law (at their own insistence) from doing the injecting. The task has fallen to technicians and other personnel.

The first such execution in Texas in 1982 was attempted by prison employees. They had great difficulty in trying to pierce the badly scarred veins of the condemned man with a large needle, and blood was spattered all over the sheets. Among those witnessing the bungled attempt was the prison doctor, who was quoted as saying that he could have done the job faster and neater. When criticized by other doctors for his remarks, he retorted that there was nothing wrong in wanting things done properly.[15]

That episode served as a warning, which the medical profession chooses to ignore: only the highest degree of technical competence should be relied upon to insure trouble-free lethal injection, to avert unnecessary suffering, and, even more important, to minimize the potential danger of inadvertent suffocation of the condemned.

There is still another good reason to insist on the highest degree of competence in performing the injections. Thiopental solution is very alkaline and therefore caustic. Accidental injection into tissue outside of a vein causes severe damage with pain (and eventual ulceration if the subject lives long enough). Furthermore, injection by mistake into an artery produces immediate and excruciating pain.

So, after all this, which method of execution is best? The choice depends on the aim in view. Lethal injection probably is the most tolerable method on a subjective level, at least in terms of anticipation. But when it comes to the technicalities of performance, the guillotine doubtlessly is easier to use, more uniformly consistent, and absolutely certain. And having an elephant squash the victim's head is the quickest of all and the surest way to eliminate the vexing question of residual consciousness.

Science really can't help us much in deciding on the one best method. In general it tends to be a selection based on common sense and an indefinable "gut" feeling. Now, admittedly this is a precarious way to deal with a profound dilemma. There is a much better way, but it will take effort.

Thus far we have been discussing only the "what" and the "how" of capital punishment. The "what" is self-explanatory. But if we are to identify the best of the "how," the best way to carry it out, then we'll have to answer the hardest question of all—the "why" of capital punishment. And that will take more than plain common sense and a "gut" feeling. That awesome obligation calls for the invocation of a uniquely human and frequently abused faculty—*ratiocination*, exact thinking applied to what society says the aim of the death penalty *should be* and what the aim *really is*.

5

Execution *Par Excellence*

It seems to be a quirk of human nature to overestimate the nobility of our achievements as well as our potential for achieving. For what other reason does every generation consider itself to be at the pinnacle of enlightenment, to be at or very close to the ideal in the agonizing evolution of what is gratuitously called civilized society?

Despite the enduring and always bitter debate over capital punishment, there is little doubt that our society today—at least those collective groups comprising "civilized humanity"—considers its attitude toward the practice to be more enlightened and closer to a perfectly ideal goal than was the case at any previous time. It is gratifying to humanitarian opponents that the death penalty now seems to be disappearing throughout the world; and equally humanitarian proponents are gratified that where vestiges persist, mollifying methods are being introduced to carry it out.

In the final analysis the debate is futile and manifests a deplorable narrowness of historical perspective. Both sides apparently ignore or reject the cyclical theory of history first postulated by the pre-Socratic philosophers and restated in our time by sages such as Nietzsche and Spengler. It is difficult to deny that human existence seems to be conditioned by some sort of cosmic, pendulumlike essence that tends to be underestimated or overlooked, particularly by those who oppose capital punishment.

I take a neutral position on the issue of capital punishment. It was, is, and probably always will be an extremely controversial and debatable topic. Any resolution will, in all likelihood, be temporary at best, and will depend not only on the sentiment (and I do mean sentiment) of those in control of government at the time but also on the prevailing social and economic conditions. Only a fool would doubt that during violent revolutions and catastrophic economic depressions the incidence of executions would skyrocket.

The "pendulum" of capital punishment is unstoppable. Its use has fluctuated throughout recorded history, and there is not an interval of peacetime during which it completely disappeared. That is potent, indeed invincible, evidence that the practice probably emanates from the very core of the human psyche and will never be eradicated.

Even the various gods invented by humankind to help face the terrifying unknowns of existence are in favor of the ultimate penalty. They not only mandate it but they even pass the death sentence on capitally sinful mortals, and serve as its executioners. Yahweh and Allah have condemned and executed millions guilty of the capital crime of lacking faith. The true believers may have been the sword, but the gods were the executioners who wielded it. In fact, they are still swinging it wildly in Lebanon, Iran, Ireland, and India.

To hope for the *permanent* abolition of judicial execution is unreasonable and unrealistic. It will always recur or be in use somewhere. That calls for the adoption of the *best* way to put it into practice, which once again brings up the problem of how to define "best." Many contemporary supporters of the death penalty would say that the best has already been achieved with the introduction of lethal injection. But clear reasoning will show that not much has really changed.

Confusion and uncertainty about the basic aim of capital punishment are at the root of the dilemma. Exactly why are capital offenders killed?

First of all to punish, of course. A capital criminal is considered to have been severely punished when his or her life is ended. Now, how can that be? Punishment means the infliction of pain or distress, either physical or mental; but a corpse can experience nothing. Punishment has no meaning for a dead person. The only possibility of punishment with regard to the death penalty can be the distress caused by the anticipation of being killed and the anxiety over the method selected to do the killing, both of which the penalty (the supposed punishment) immediately relieves! We have here the nonsensical paradox of a supreme punishment that punishes only if it is not inflicted.

Then there is the question of deterrence. Opponents are fond of citing statistics to support their contention that the death penalty has very little to do with preventing capital crime. Contrarily, those in favor of capital punishment interpret the statistics differently; their rebuttal seems to be that if deterrence can't be proved, neither can it be disproved. At present the consensus is that the matter is unsettled at best. But one can therefore hardly insist on deterrence being the primary aim of the death penalty.

An aim perpetually at the top of society's list is "retribution." This euphemism for "revenge" is a big part of the problem. Originally the word retribution meant compensation or something of value given in return. How can the involuntary death of a criminal fit that definition? What is returned to society or to anyone in it? There can be no compensation from executions as traditionally understood; there can be only loss of life.

In the final analysis capital punishment can have only two definite and absolutely unarguable aims. The first is simply to put an end to a criminal's earthly existence. The second is to prevent repetition of crime by the individual thus eliminated. Debating any other ultimately unprovable aim can only further muddy the already murky waters of furious and unending controversy.

Unfortunately something theoretically irrefutable—in this case the unarguable aims of the death penalty—can be subverted by clever hypocrisy. That has always been true in this ugly realm of human behavior in which high-sounding but insincere philosophizing obscures the real motive underlying most, if not all, judicial killing: plain revenge, and frequently the more brutal and agonizing the better. In that way an otherwise elusive (and certainly unjustifiable) aim is achieved: the "punishment" of guaranteed physical and mental anguish deceitfully rationalized as "inadvertent" or "unintended" before the victim becomes an unfeeling corpse.

Is our contemporary way of dealing with capital punishment the most enlightened ever devised? The question is unanswered because we have looked at only the *physical* aspect of the purposeful destruction of human life, and that may be the least important aspect. We have to consider the abstract components, too. Only they can prove whether the aims of the death penalty are noble enough to be worthy of the human spirit, and only they can be the true arbiters of the inherent value of those aims.

All of the methods of execution thus far have but one purpose: to end a criminal's physical existence, in what is hoped to be the most humane way possible. The only abstraction thereby honored is secular law. That certainly is a noble aim, but *how* noble when that entirely *artificial* abstraction is compared with other totally ignored but even more meaningful and much more fundamental *natural* abstractions? After all, artificial law is a mere invention of the natural human mind, which itself is the essence of the natural human spirit.

Therefore, the execution of a human being should aim far higher than simply to satisfy the law. Such an epochal event should serve as a means of elucidating the what, why, and how of human thought and action—especially those of a criminal nature—and of health and disease, and of life and death. In contrast to invented law, these are all inscrutable, preexistent phenomena of nature arbitrarily (and ineptly) conceptualized by man. And without them no other invention, abstract or concrete, could exist, let alone have value.

Herein lies the perpetual tragedy of capital punishment. The progress purportedly made in the humane technique of its physical implementation pales to insignificance in the face of this glaring deficiency in its theoretical framework. The puny advance that lethal injection might be said to represent from a physical standpoint cannot begin to balance the abysmal spiritual void it nevertheless sustains. In and of itself lethal injection cannot reverse the retrogression manifested in the way we sacrifice human beings to appease the minor deity of abstract law alone.

What is the proof of this retrogression—that we are not only *not* marking time, but also actually retreating from some sort of superior code of conduct? Recorded history offers two proofs, one somewhat problematical, the other definite.

As mentioned earlier, the first probably prevailed in Ptolemaic Alexandria around the third century B.C. Here was the high point of ancient civilization that fostered an atmosphere of unbridled thought and investigation unequalled, even in our time. Science and art flourished under enlightened rulers who encouraged men of genius. In this exciting scenario, according to Roman historians, the kings were supposed to have decreed that since condemned criminals owed society a huge debt, they were to be executed in anatomical laboratories.

Although conclusive evidence is lacking, many historians believe that execution for medical purposes was practiced in that golden age of research. Having lasted for only three centuries, that age witnessed the first attempt to tap the strictly spiritual aspect of capital punishment by using it to probe the aforementioned natural abstractions, which are far more important and deserving than law.

But retrogression set in when the hegemony of Rome stripped executions of the high aims imbued by the Alexandrians. The retrogression continued into the cistern which was the Dark Ages. Then another reversal occurred, astonishingly, with the incipient Renaissance, and, amazingly, in the Armenia of Asia Minor. I learned of that extraordinary episode only in 1987. According to a report in an obscure foreign-language newspaper, the medieval Armenians were doing exactly what the Alexandrians had supposedly done a millennium and a half earlier. They were subjecting condemned criminals to medical experiments during execution.

I verified this from articles published recently in academic journals from Soviet Armenia (see chapter 10). These articles, in turn, cited publications in the classical Armenian language from around 1350 to 1375 describing the practice then in vogue. They also tended to verify what I had guessed about Alexandria: experiments were performed there only after subjects were rendered insensitive with large amounts of alcohol. Much of the Armenian research dealt with observation of organ structure and function, including circulation of the blood. This then represents the second and well-documented episode of man's homage to the nobler and usually ignored values inherent in the willful destruction of humans.

The backsliding of modern society in this regard is obvious. We wantonly squander priceless opportunities to study ourselves and our living brains, as well as new ways to make us wiser, healthier, and happier. Worse yet, in our "most enlightened" way of serving justice, we don't even *think* about making the attempt. So we sanctimoniously keep snuffing out the lives of criminals, many of whom acknowledge their transgression and sincerely desire to somehow make amends. They are eager to give society *real* retribution by donating their organs and by helping science unlock some of nature's deepest secrets by submitting to otherwise impossible experimentation.

But society will not allow it, and doctors refuse to accept it. In callously overriding the personal autonomy of the condemned by denying them the privilege of choice, we inflict on them the worst kind of suffering—far more agonizing than any physical pain—the crushing pain of a tortured mind and a turbulent soul denied any hope of requital.

This is forcefully driven home in a recent letter to me written by a fifty-year-old inmate awaiting electrocution on Georgia's death row: "It's cruel . . . to deny me the chance to donate my organs and make that degree of restitution. I am forced to meet my maker having taken a life and being denied the chance to give life to people so desperately in need. *I am forced to exit this world with a troubled heart and anxious mind*" (italics added).

That is the ultimate proof of retrogression. It is why we delude ourselves when we insist that our way, this generation's handling of judicial executions, is the most enlightened.

6

Bad News from Sacramento

It was late in the morning of 23 April 1984 when I arrived by bus at the entrance of San Quentin Prison. While the guard at the gate stepped into his booth to check credentials, I took in the panorama of neat buildings evenly spread out over spacious and well-kept grounds. Here and there among the buildings prisoners worked calmly and guards walked slowly. It was in stark contrast to the foreboding high stone walls at the old Ohio Penitentiary in Columbus, and, of course, less intimidating after twenty-eight years of experience. Within minutes I was walking past prisoners, busy at their landscaping chores, toward the administration building and the warden's reception room.

Unlike the informality in Columbus, here I had to conform to strict regulations regarding permission for death row interviews. However, there was much more involved here than my desire to question an inmate; that's why I had no difficulty obtaining permission.

My visit was prompted—almost mandated—by the pending hearing on Senate Bill SB 1968, for which I was to testify that afternoon in Sacramento.

The chain of events leading to that hearing began in January 1984. When I learned that a member of the Judiciary Committee of the California Senate was considering the substitution of lethal drug injection for the gas chamber as the official method of execution, I wrote to him to suggest that any such contemplated legislation incorporate a choice for the donation of organs. The senator referred my suggestion to a colleague on the Judiciary Committee, who also happened to be a member of the select legislative committee concerned with anatomical transplants. A couple of weeks later I was overjoyed to learn from the colleague's aide that he had acknowledged the merit of the idea and was preparing an appropriate bill.

There was no doubt that my testimony would be crucial. I put together all the supporting evidence I had on hand, including copies of a couple of letters from death row. But these inmates were in other states. For maximum impact and credibility I needed comments from California's death row. Surely, I thought, that alone would be enough to convince the committee members to bring the bill before the full senate. With this kind of implied legislative imprimatur behind my request, Warden Dan Vasquez cordially and quickly granted me permission to interview five death row inmates on the morning of 23 April. That would leave me enough time to get to Sacramento for the afternoon hearing loaded with opinions fresh from inmates' mouths.

Several copies of the proposed bill had been sent to me about three weeks before the scheduled hearing (figure 2). It seemed that at last the concept was about to come up for public debate, if not to be actually implemented. My excitement grew when a morning newscast on a local radio station mentioned the forthcoming hearing a few days before it was to take place. But later that day I had my first doubts. Usually such news items are repeated frequently throughout the day, particularly if the station had an all-news format. This one wasn't repeated—which should have tipped me off that something unforeseen had happened.

SENATE BILL   No. 1968

Introduced by Senator Speraw

February 16, 1984

An act to amend Section 3604 of the Penal Code, relating to execution.

LEGISLATIVE COUNSEL'S DIGEST

SB 1968, as introduced, Speraw. Execution.

Existing law requires infliction of the death penalty by administration of lethal gas.

This bill would require the Director of Corrections to provide an alternative method of execution in cases in which the subject has provided for donation upon death of organs or tissues under the Uniform Anatomical Gift Act.

Vote: majority. Appropriation: no. Fiscal committee: yes. State-mandated local program: no.

The people of the State of California do enact as follows:

1   SECTION 1. Section 3604 of the Penal Code is
2 amended to read:
3   3604. *(a)* The punishment of death shall be inflicted
4 by the administration of a lethal gas.
5   *(b) Notwithstanding subdivision (a), the Legislature*
6 *finds and declares that the administration of lethal gas*
7 *effectively negates the purpose and intent of the Uniform*
8 *Anatomical Gift Act by making human organs and tissues*
9 *so exposed unacceptable for medical transplant purposes.*
10 *Therefore, an alternative method of execution which is*
11 *determined by the Director of Corrections to minimize*
12 *damage to organs and tissue shall be provided in any case*
13 *in which the subject has provided for the donation upon*
14 *death of his or her organs or tissue in accordance with the*
15 *Uniform Anatomical Gift Act.*

O

99 60

Figure 2. California Senate Bill 1968 (April 1984)

The bad news struck on the warm and sunny morning of 22 April. The windows of my apartment were wide open, and I heard mail being delivered to my box. I fetched it, and the first thing I spotted was a small notice that an overnight registered letter had to be signed for. Why hadn't the mailman rung the doorbell? I had to know what was in that letter before leaving for San Quentin very early the next morning. I rushed out to search for the mailman. Fortunately I caught up with him around the corner, and with relief I signed for the letter.

It was from the committee chairman's office in Sacramento. My doubts hardened as I opened the envelope and began reading the letter dated 20 April (!):

> I was unable to reach you today but wanted to let you know what the senator plans to do about SB 1968 re: alternative method for execution. Earlier this week this office met with the representatives of the Department of Corrections. They are opposing this measure because of the adverse effects it would have on the future of any execution in California. This administration is very interested in seeing the will of California citizens implemented.
>
> But SB 1968 is providing an alternative method when California does not even institute its death penalty. Another reason for opposition is the numbers of transplants would not be that great with death row inmates. The real figures are with the total prison population.
>
> As a result this office plans to cooperate with the administration in implementing a donor awareness program within California's prison system. We will therefore be dropping SB 1968 from our legislative file.
>
> I apologize for any inconvenience this might have caused you, but I honestly believe this approach will be a more favorable one for the organ donor program.
>
> (Signed by the senator's aide)

I was angry and disappointed. Why didn't they call me with such vital news instead of sending it though the mail? It would have been much more considerate. After all, two full days had elapsed since the decision was made and the belated letter sent. And those illogical reasons for dropping the bill—none of them could stand up against the counterarguments flashing through my mind.

There should have been no connection between my proposal and any existing organ donor program. I had previously contacted transplant teams in the United States and knew that they wouldn't get involved in organ procurement during executions. Therefore, death row donation could never be a part of any organized system. But that doesn't justify ignoring priceless organs simply because their source is distinct from, and alien to, the conventional realm of medical practice and societal tradition. To a dying patient this is totally irrational and downright cruel.

The incredible objection that death row wouldn't supply enough organs to be worth bothering about was even harder for me to stomach. It signified the senator's failure (or refusal) to grasp the main thrust of my proposal. It is not the quantitative effects of the death penalty that count, but rather the *quality* of the act. As currently practiced its effects are zero at best, but certainly tending toward the negative.

First, the death of the condemned simply compounds the victim's loss of life. Add to this the even more sickening loss of several lives when salvageable patients die waiting for innocent donor organs, which are already in critically short supply. The crucial element is not the number of lives that might be saved, but rather the *attempt* to impart some kind of indisputably positive value to the purposeful extinction of human life.

As I pointed out in chapter 5, the essence, or quality, of the death penalty has always been misconstrued. It has centered very narrowly on the physical means used and their surmised effect on the body being killed. The only positive aspect of capital punishment—as conventionally understood—is its attempt to satisfy justice. Everything else connected with judicial execution is irrevocable loss. So, anything that diminishes, or merely strives to diminish, loss can only enhance the quality of the act. Therefore, the taking of organs from just *one* condemned criminal a year, or from one per decade, enhances the quality or essence of capital punishment. That would still be true if only a single kidney were culled and used; or even if, for some reason, that solitary kidney couldn't be used.

Numbers have little to do with the morality of an act. The determining factors are the intent of the actor(s) and the significance of the real or putative consequences of acting. It is equally immoral for someone to murder one human being or ten.

The matter boils down to honoring a condemned person's right of choice to permit the harvesting of life from death. *That* is the way to enhance the quality of capital punishment; and that is my primary aim. Everything else, such as how many condemned prisoners will go along with it and how many organs will be obtained, are questions of secondary importance and, in fact, irrelevant.

It was difficult for me to believe that the senator seriously hoped to get many organs from the thousands of noncondemned prisoners in the state. That seemed silly because voluntary organ donation on the part of today's prisoners is a vain idea. The exploitation of prison populations has been anathema since the sensational abuses and corruption in connection with drug research on prisoners in the 1950s and 1960s. Furthermore, bioethicists claim that consent by prisoners is never freely given, but rather is subtly coerced or financially induced. But even if it were possible, and if the entire prison population were willing to donate, what could each inmate offer but a single kidney? It would hardly be morally defensible to take one kidney from a willing noncondemned prisoner and, at the same time, condone the senseless waste of two kidneys, two lungs, a heart, a liver, a pancreas, and perhaps even intestines—all in superb biological condition—when a willing condemned prisoner is executed.

No, Senator, you dodged the issue. Other sources of organs, no matter how plentiful, are totally irrelevant. Even if the nation were flooded with a surplus of donors (which is inconceivable for the near future, at least), morality dictates that those offered by contrite condemned men and women should be used and not destroyed. After all, they owe the greatest debt to society and should have priority over any other donor, imprisoned or free. In other words, maximum indebtedness coupled with altruism is a more cogent factor than altruism alone.

SB 1968 acknowledged the truth of that. But in the senator's opinion the new method of execution was too "radical" a change at a time when capital punishment already was a nettlesome topic. He evidently agreed with officials of the Corrections Department that such a change would complicate and delay the implementation of the California's existing death penalty statute.

Was the senator worried that the change might evoke public indignation and antagonism? Perhaps; but the public was totally unaware of my proposal. Yet, even if that was his worry, it was contrary to what I had learned from many friends and strangers. By a large majority they endorsed as plain common sense the use of organs from, and even experimentation on, willing condemned criminals. Indeed, a few would go so far as to deny them the privilege of choice, saying that it subverted the concept of payment of an enormous social debt. I felt that the senator had reacted politically, not rationally.

The aide's disconcerting letter raised many specious arguments crying out for rebuttal, and I planned to write a terse response later in the day. I recalled that I had telephoned four local doctors about a month earlier to ask their opinions. They were members of the regional organ transplant council. All four gave oral approval, even though one opposed capital punishment. However, nurse coordinators for organ procurement at two major university medical schools in California denounced my proposal. One did so entirely on her own, emphatically and harshly excoriating SB 1968 as well as the proposal in general. The other nurse merely conveyed the decision of surgeons with whom she had discussed the matter: the surgeons would take organs only from clinically brain-dead donors in hospitals. I then asked if they would endorse SB 1968 for the benefit of other surgeons who might be willing to participate. She replied that they "would have to study the matter more thoroughly."

Members of transplant teams obviously are in close contact with state legislators serving on relevant committees. It is natural for me to suspect that pressure exerted by the transplanters was significant if not decisive in compelling the senator to withdraw his bill.

At least I could be thankful that I had intercepted the registered letter in time to avert an unnecessary detour to Sacramento. Despite my disappointment I would go to San Quentin anyway to take advantage of a rare opportunity.

That afternoon I wrote the senator's aide, indicating that I felt somewhat betrayed by the sudden death of his bill. I summarized my feelings in the last paragraph: "At any rate I appreciated the senator's evanescent interest, even if it was for what I consider to be the wrong reasons. He has passed up a unique chance to make a mark in the history of humanism, but evidently the price was too high."

I mailed my reply, returned home to relax and to retire early. But sleep didn't come easily, as I eagerly anticipated my pre-dawn bus ride to San Quentin the following morning and the extraordinary experience awaiting me there.

7

Voices from Death Row

Shortly before 11:00 A.M. I entered the warden's reception room and was greeted by his assistant. Warden Dan Vasquez entered about five minutes later, and the three of us casually discussed the reason for my visit. The warden's comments were terse, general, and noncommittal. I was then escorted by his assistant to a very large, pleasant, wood-paneled room that was completely bare except for several plain chairs and a large wooden table. I was allowed to use only a pen and a pad of paper to jot down notes during the interviews, which were witnessed by the assistant.

Two of the inmates had changed their minds about talking to me. Each of the remaining three was brought in alone and seated opposite me at the table. There was no time limit. And for the sake of objectivity it was my decision to keep from knowing the inmates' names, the reasons for their imprisonment, or anything about their personal histories.

While waiting for the assistant to bring the first man, I reflected on how much more secure and confident I felt when compared to my first death row experience in Columbus a quarter-century earlier. Mine was still a one-man campaign, to be sure; and the concept was still quite obscure and far from public knowledge. But to me it was like an infant, no longer newborn, growing slowly but now steadily, with impeccable birth credentials and a gradually widening circle of intimate admirers. I had, by now, committed myself to nurturing it to robust adulthood—and entirely by myself if need be. I viewed these interviews as supplying some of the required nutriment.

The first man was a well-built Caucasian of average height, who appeared somewhat younger looking than his forty-four years, and without any distinguishing facial features. After an exchange of the usual polite greetings, I thanked him for volunteering to talk with me. He had a good command of language and a fairly high degree of intelligence. I came straight to the point: would he prefer to die in the gas chamber, as is now stipulated by law, or have a choice of being put to death by general anesthesia so that his organs could be taken for transplantation? Without hesitation he emphatically opted for anesthesia.

It soon became apparent why his reply had been so quick and definite. Even before having heard of me or my campaign, on his own he had been involved in legal proceedings to force transplant surgeons at Stanford University to take his organs if and when he were executed. It didn't surprise me that his efforts had been in vain. Nevertheless he insisted that he would continue to press his request in trying to avoid what he adamantly decried as "a waste of human life."

Those were mighty pleasing words to me. But I wondered if he knew what he was talking about when he spoke of anesthesia. Had he undergone general anesthesia for some kind of surgical procedure? His opinion would be unassailable only if he knew first-hand exactly all that the experience involved. I was relieved to hear him mention eight previous operations, seven on a knee, one on a thumb; and he had experienced general anesthesia induced by a relatively fast-acting barbiturate given intravenously. He emphasized that he knew for sure the superiority of anesthesia as a way to put a man to death and, at the same time, make it possible for others to live from the transplanted organs. He placed no limit on the number of organs to be harvested from his execution.

Even more gratifying was his attitude with regard to my original idea of experimentation on anesthetized condemned individuals. Here, too, he placed no limits. Researchers could perform any experiments they deemed useful on any part of his anesthetized body, including deep probes into the most sensitive areas of the brain and central nervous system. New and previously untried drugs could be tested for their effects, which might eventually prove to be valuable, he said. To gain one tiny new fact from such an execution would be better than simply destroying a human life for the social satisfaction of exacting revenge. This was the kind of broad, inflinching, and unconditional support my "infant" idea needed.

I was stunned by his advanced thinking. What was the wellspring of his opinion? Was it purely a personal decision? Or did extraneous factors come into play? I asked if concern for his own family members or consideration of the victim of his crime or of the victim's family had anything to do with his conclusions. He retorted, "Absolutely none!" This unadorned response took me by surprise, but I would later learn that it is a common attitude among condemned convicts.

This inmate claimed to be well known among other prisoners as a competent and completely self-taught legal adviser. He claimed to be aware of everything that was going on among them. He assured me that many noncondemned prisoners prefer death by lethal injection to life forever behind bars. This opinion was confirmed by the results of a poll I took later that year, and by extensive correspondence with a convict in federal prison who was waging his own campaign to have the option legalized.

Five minutes after the first convict left the room, the second condemned man was ushered in. He, too, was Caucasian and appeared to be younger than his stated age of forty. For him death by anesthesia was preferable to death in the gas chamber, and he was in favor of his organs being taken. As he put it: "There are many people in need, and that way I wouldn't be dying for nothing." But he rejected the idea of experimentation while under anesthesia. Nevertheless, I had the feeling that with further, purely objective discussion he would have consented. But I didn't want to risk even appearing to persuade or plead a case during these interviews.

In contrast to the surgical experiences of the first inmate interviewed, this man had been operated on only for a tonsillectomy and had never been anesthetized by injection of a barbiturate. Again in contrast, he said that his family would approve of, and feel better about, his decision to donate organs. But what the reactions of the victim's family might be were, he said, of absolutely no importance or consequence with regard to his decision.

His remarkable insight and unsolicited advice reinforced my plan of attack. I was pleased to hear him suggest that the best route for my proposal was to arouse public support to petition legislators and pressure them into changing the law. Evidently he already knew what took me a while to learn, namely, that the average citizen would view my proposal as a very common-sense solution to a knotty problem, and not at all as the terrifying bugaboo it seemed to be to politicians. The sagacious inmate even advised me to try to bring along a few legislators on future visits to death row.

I recognized that the ultimate key to success was right there on death row, and he himself was part of it. Only the very loud and persistent voices of those who really count—those who by the very nature of their circumstances are sincere and must be taken seriously—would be powerful enough to arouse public opinion. I realized that this is the one force politicians would never dare oppose and cannot long resist.

The third condemned man was a youthful, good looking, light complexioned twenty-seven-year-old African-American of short stature. His placid demeanor and calm, almost whispered voice belied a touch of mental depression, the cause of which soon became apparent. He emphatically endorsed both medical aspects of my proposal. "Surgeons can take all of my organs," he said, "because people need them." In addition, he would submit to unrestricted medical experimentation because "there's a great need for research, and it could possibly save many lives," he explained. His only experience with general anesthesia was inhaling ether for a tonsillectomy.

He also surprised me by revealing that he had already inquired about being accepted as an organ donor. I then began to realize that the sense of altruism or meaningful contrition is more prevalent on death row than most people might guess, or most authorities (especially medical authorities) would care to acknowledge.

This inmate cared a great deal about what his relatives thought. He stated with subdued satisfaction that he preferred death by lethal injection to lifelong incarceration. In his low-key fashion he complained bitterly about the complete lack of privacy and the unrelenting, highly irritating noise of an overcrowded prison. For him that brief interview in a large, quiet room offered a rare respite from the maddening cacophony. He lamented the seeming unfairness of having committed only one crime in his lifetime, for which society had placed him among brutal men to await a meaningless end to his life.

But he concluded on a firm note. He said he hoped that his wish for a useful death would not be thwarted by those who are against my proposal because they oppose the death penalty. "They do not help me," he continued, "when they say that you are barbaric and wrong."

Finally, in order to silence disingenuous critics, I asked if I had intimidated or pressured him during our discourse. He replied that his opinions and decisions were freely given and were not conditioned by stressful circumstances (as those who reject my proposal would have us believe).

The interview ended at 12:50 P.M. I leaned back with satisfaction as the warden's assistant escorted the docile inmate out of the room. It had been a tremendously productive two hours. Especially noteworthy among all three inmates was their courteous and friendly attitudes, their articulate speech, and their forthright and seemingly honest responses. Another common trait was their apparent lack of fear of death. What troubled them most was the prospect of a pointless death. The same sentiment prevailed in many letters I received from death row inmates in other states over the next several years.

Back in the reception room I thanked the warden and his assistant. As I walked toward the gate to await the bus for my return to Long Beach, elation over what I had accomplished at San Quentin expunged the disappointment caused by the negative letter from the senator's aide. I was now more convinced than ever that it was futile to seek a solution at the top, so to speak.

The route to take was from the bottom up, as two of the interviewed inmates had suggested. Only by marshaling the strident voices from death row into a thundering chorus could I ever pierce the public's consciousness and make sure that the ignominious fate of SB 1968 would never be repeated.

The long afternoon bus ride back to Long Beach was ideal for mapping out my strategy. What I lacked in power and resources was more than compensated for by the unshakable conviction that what I was trying to accomplish was unquestionably right. And it will always be right as long as medicine is practiced and human beings are judicially destroyed.

Despite the loud and angry denunciation from my opponents, I had no doubt that deep down in their psyche they, too, knew that it is right. Therefore, it really didn't matter what I said or how I said it; there was actually no need for persuasion. As a guide there was my own personal experience which, combined with the thoughts of past savants, was enough to convince me that acceptance and implementation of my proposal hinged on more than my most strenuous efforts or those of any other individual. I finally had to admit what my puerile exuberance tried to deny: ideas succeed not primarily because they are proclaimed, but because their time has come.

I had suspected that as far back as 1960 and reluctantly said so in an article entitled "The Nobler Execution" in the literary journal *Ararat*. It soon became evident the time was not ripe: a moratorium on the death penalty in the United States went into effect in the late 1960s and early 1970s, and my campaign ground to a virtual standstill. I didn't reactivate it until the resumption of executions in the mid-1970s—and only then in a low-key way, even though death rows throughout the county were rapidly becoming crowded.

Then something unexpected happened. Combined with the gathering momentum for capital punishment, it helped ripen the time for my proposal. The unexpected boon was the rapid evolution of whole organ transplantation to almost routine and daily surgical practice.

The idea of unrestricted medical experimentation on willing, doomed criminals might still seem to be "barbaric" and "cruel" to my detractors, I reasoned. But common sense could not be stretched to justify denying criminals the privilege (or right) of donating organs when they die, to assure that certain patients could live. It was that simple. It was beyond doubt. It was time to act—23 April 1984!

My intention to contact men on death row actually had grown out of the interest and initial action in the California senator's office three months earlier. To avoid or minimize criticism that the topic would be unduly provocative or bothersome for prisoners already in the stressful milieu of death row, I decided to write only to those whose names cropped up in newspaper stories, whose executions were imminent, and whose appeals had been rejected by the United States Supreme Court. I felt that these prisoners might look upon my proposal as a last, if futile, glimmer of hope. At first I had mistakenly assumed that every rejected appeal was the last one. I soon learned that a condemned convict may exhaust as many as nine appeals extending over many years before execution.

For one of the first inmates I had written to, in January 1984, my proposal was indeed a glimmer of hope. Fred Dorsey* faced electrocution in Michigan City, Indiana. Before receiving my letter, he had decided to forgo all appeals. In his reply he lamented the state's refusal to legitimate lethal injection as an execution option, and he doubted that what a condemned man said could have much influence or value in that regard.

But he did endorse my proposal, with these words: "Every breath

---

*An asterisk next to a proper name denotes the use of a fictitious name in order to avoid jeopardizing an inmate's appeal or tenuous legal situation.

I take is more than my victims will *ever* take, and their families know this. . . . That is an additional form of grief to them. I don't like to make people sad, and I have done some horrible things. I *owe* my life but at least should be able to go in a way I choose. . . . Perhaps my family could really accept my death if they felt that some good will come of it."

At his request I telephoned Dorsey about two weeks later, and the real "glimmer of hope" was evident. He had thought it over and decided to begin the appeals process to gain time in a fight for lethal injection. This unexpected result was especially pleasing: it contradicted a criticism, widespread among my opponents, that the concept would heap more psychological stress upon an already burdened prisoner.

Three months later, shortly before my trip to San Quentin, inmate Arthur Bishop wrote me the following from his cell on death row in Draper, Utah: "When I know that my death is immediate and inevitable, I would gladly arrange for the donation of my organs and would also allow, if possible, such medical experimentation. . . . Perhaps in doing this my death could offer some partial atonement for my crimes. . . . I feel that all condemned men should be allowed to determine the method of their death if they desire to donate their organs. If I must die, let me die believing that my death may give some benefit to someone or that some medical gain may be achieved. Let my final act bring about some good rather than just serving as an appeasement of society's need for revenge."

We exchanged several more letters over the next fourteen months. In these Bishop collaborated on the poll I conducted in the summer of 1984. He volunteered to distribute my questionnaire among a few others on Utah's death row and to return the completed forms. I tabulated the results and submitted them to the international journal *Medicine and Law* for publication in 1985.[3] Later Bishop wrote that he would be concentrating on his appeals over the following two or three years. I didn't contact him again until 1987—just a brief note to inquire how things were going. My letter was returned unopened.

When the same attempt was repeated and returned in the early summer of 1988, I realized that something drastic had happened. My first suspicion was that corrections officials probably thwarted his wish to donate organs. But a hurried and stern letter to the Utah Corrections Department proved me wrong. The state, by that time, had instituted the option of lethal injection; I was told in no uncertain terms that Bishop had indeed been given the privilege of choosing to donate organs but had changed his mind and refused. He died by lethal drug injection in June 1985.

It seems that Bishop's main objective was simply to assure a more tolerable mode of death. And even though his original support of my campaign might have been less than honest or purely altruistic, the episode proved several things. First, a condemned individual's autonomy of choice must be respected at all times. Second, any initial assent must be firm and unwavering. Third, the right to reverse that assent must be guaranteed. And finally, anyone who manifests uncertainty or has a change of heart after consenting must never again be a candidate for organ donation or experimentation.

Not long after the San Quentin interviews, I spotted a news item about another condemned murderer, housed at the same institution, who also wanted to dispense with all appeals and be executed as soon as possible. Jerry Bigelow's situation was almost identical to that of Dorsey. In a newspaper article Bigelow was described as a blue-eyed, clean-cut, well-behaved twenty-four-year-old wearing number 55 on death row since 1981. He and another death row resident (perhaps one of those I had interviewed earlier) were self-taught and quite knowledgeable in law, and were working through official channels to gain the right to be executed without delay. I wrote to Bigelow, who had freely admitted to reporters that he had committed cold-blooded murder, details of which he nonchalantly described. The prospect of being put to death bothered him less than the incessant noise and disagreeable odors of prison life.

We corresponded for about a year, but there was no telephone contact, and we never met personally. The reasons for his solid support of both organ donation and experimentation are clearly stated in his letters: "The result I hope for is that people will not only realize that the condemned . . . are not all bad; but also to show that unless we, the condemned, are executed with this new-found purpose being in existence, then the death penalty is not out to serve the ultimate good of society in practical ways, but serve only the lesser, more base emotions of a society bent on revenge. I only hope that I am able to make my points . . . known to the general public."

Taking another cynical swipe at society's current attitude, Bigelow continued: "The death penalty is now controlled by people who are bent on vengeance . . . (so) why not subvert their intentions by introducing aspects like organ donation and thiopental which are . . . one step removed from vengeance and pain and one step closer to kindness, and thereby corrupt them with a bit of decency." What astounding rhetoric from death row!

Lest his real motives be misunderstood, in another letter Bigelow admitted that he was not concerned "about repaying society or (about) my influence in making historic changes. I am not motivated by pious ideology either. I would like to assure you that my reason for doing things that may bring about the use of lethal injection . . . is completely self-serving."

Among those things he did was to distribute my questionnaire where possible and to encourage those within his reach to take part. Interest had already been stimulated by word of my interviews several weeks before. I was unaware of the fact that on their own he and twenty-eight other condemned men had prepared and signed a petition demanding the option of lethal injection in lieu of lethal gas for those who wanted to donate organs. I received this valuable document in July 1984 and have made good use of it since (see Appendix).

It was with mixed feelings that I read Bigelow's last letter informing me that his conviction had been overturned and that he had been transferred to a county jail to await a new trial. On the one hand, I could not lament his good luck in having escaped, even if only temporarily, the torturous din of a state penitentiary and the bleak fate of a degrading execution. But on the other hand, I had lost the credible voice of an ardent and sincere advocate.

New support was to be found in material published by two noncondemned prisoners. David Holdaway was a budding author nearing the end of his imprisonment in the Federal Penitentiary at Lompoc, California. In an erudite essay published in the Cleveland *Plain Dealer* on 6 April 1984, Holdaway supported the death penalty as being merciful as well as educational. "In my time in custody," he wrote, "I have seen dozens of men for whom capital punishment would be a godsend. Trudging blankly from cellblock to dining hall to work assignment day after day, month after month, year after year, their sentences are a weight which has crushed the life out of them, reducing them to shuffling lumps of angry protoplasm."

In his reply to me Holdaway heartily endorsed organ donation, but he had reservations about experimentation and chose to remain neutral. All the other prisoners to whom he showed my material agreed with organ donation, but their responses to the choice for experiments, he wrote, ranged "all over the spectrum."

It was Holdaway's personal feeling "that either should be an option. If a condemned man wishes to donate organs, fine. If he agrees to medical experimentation, fine, too. If both are okay with him, that's okay with me." What refreshing rationality, toleration, and common sense! If only the authorities in control of society's pertinent institutions, especially those concerned with health care, were similarly disposed.

The second source of support was fifty-four-year-old James Carey, who came to my attention through his letter to the editor of the Los Angeles *Herald Examiner* on 10 March 1984, one of many newspapers throughout the nation to which this letter had been sent. Having already served two very unpleasant years of a fifty-year sentence in the federal penitentiary at Terre Haute, Indiana, Carey pleaded for the option of death by lethal injection. He asked that it be granted to any inmate facing long-term incarceration under conditions he or she deemed to be torturous and intolerable. Because Carey's campaign was relevant to mine, I wrote to solicit his opinion.

It did not surprise me that he responded with enthusiasm. He made his endorsement explicit in a subsequent letter to members of Congress, which was entered into the *Congressional Record* of 8 May 1984: "We would gladly accept death by lethal injection and donate our bodies to medical science in lieu of enduring interminable degradation. Therefore, I appeal to you to introduce or lend support to legislation that would grant any defendant sentenced to serve over three years imprisonment in the federal penal system the option of a voluntary death sentence."

These two federal prisoners also cooperated in distributing the questionnaire I was circulating at the time. Because the appeal for an optional death sentence was inextricably linked to my campaign, I included a question about the acceptability of that choice. Both men participated and persuaded other inmates to join in.

The questionnaire consisted of seventeen relatively simple items that focused on capital punishment, methods of execution, the respondents' previous experience with anesthesia, and their opinions regarding my proposed medical options. All responses were anonymous in order to encourage participation and to enhance honesty. Originally the questionnaire was intended for condemned prisoners only, but Carey's project required the inclusion of other convicts. That led to further expansion and eventually to the sampling of a more general cross section of society.

With the cooperation of two professors at California State University Long Beach, two classrooms of undergraduate students in psychology and sociology were asked to take part. I also wanted to test adolescents at the local high school but was denied permission by the Long Beach Board of Education. Finally, because medical opposition was so obstinate and emotional, it was only with trepidation (and almost as an afterthought) that I queried medical personnel at five hospitals, including two affiliated with medical schools.

The results from both groups of prisoners were astonishing. Over a third of the condemned men and three-fourths of other prisoners favored the broadest choice of either organ donation or experimentation. And almost half of the condemned opted for organ donation at least. Even more surprising was the endorsement of capital punishment itself by slightly less than half of the condemned and, again, three-fourths of the noncondemned inmates. The fear of death wasn't much of a factor for either group. And the results also confirmed Jerry Bigelow's frank admission that the offer of medical benefits "is completely self-serving" and essentially devoid of an altruistic concern for others. In general, any ostensible altruism is self-directed as though aimed at ameliorating or rectifying an intuitively perceived moral defect.

It seems almost incredible that the same may be true for those on the receiving end of capital crime. In 1984, I interviewed in their home near Los Angeles the parents of a fourteen-year-old boy who had been murdered approximately a year earlier. The killer was on San Quentin's death row, and I wanted to know how the bereaved parents felt about his donating organs instead of being gassed to death. From the beginning neither parent showed enthusiasm for the possibility. The victim's mother was emotional and at times tearful; she seemed to care for nothing but the self-satisfaction of plain revenge. Whereas she kept ignoring my tactful persistence for her opinion on organ donation, as the discussion wore on, her husband appeared to accept the idea. I sensed that he was careful to avoid overt endorsement out of respect for his wife's strong feelings as well as to assuage in some measure his own powerful (and understandable) lust for revenge.

On a personal level the dilemma faced by victims' relatives and condemned killers is shared by society at large: the difficult choice between emotionally gratifying behavior on the one hand, and less satisfactory, rational behavior on the other. In other words, the conflict between what one *wants* to do and what one *ought* to do.

As mentioned earlier, data from the questionnaire were incorporated into an article published in *Medicine and Law*, an international journal based in Israel. The editor had previously accepted another of my papers which several American journal editors had rejected as being too controversial or unworthy of consideration. Again, I knew from experience that, contrary to what they avow, editors of so-called prestigious medical journals do not permit their publications to serve as open forums for ideas that they deem to be too "hot" to handle, not befitting the carefully nurtured public image of the profession, or contrary to their official journal policies. So, rather than waste time and effort grappling hypocrisy at home, I trusted that honest open-mindedness still prevailed in other countries. And I wasn't disappointed.

In the spring of 1987, I wrote to Leland Heitsch* who was condemned to electrocution at Atmore, Alabama. In his reply Heitsch stated a desire to donate organs if and when the opportunity were made available. In fact, he looked into the possibility of being a donor even before execution.

His next letter, seventeen months later, was equally supportive but more pessimistic. "Yes," he wrote, "I still support your ideas and your work. The states seem to have no reservation or hesitation to execute someone, but they want to inject the morality standard upon your idea. That in itself reeks of hypocrisy and smacks of contradiction. My efforts to become an organ donor prior to my execution have been stonewalled at every turn. They consider my idea ghoulish but embrace the concept of burning someone alive in the electric chair. Even the A.C.L.U. has shown no interest in assisting my endeavor."

The following month Heitsch named three others on death row who also supported my campaign and were ready to participate in any media event arranged to advance it. However, their attorneys advised against it for the time being in order to safeguard pending and planned appeals.

Nevertheless, I still could fall back on several advantageous contacts made in the autumn of 1988. One was in connection with the pending execution by lethal injection of twenty-eight-year-old Donald King,* scheduled for 1 December at Deer Lodge, Montana. His case was of special interest because King had already requested permission to donate organs. I wrote him a letter of encouragement and asked his opinion on my proposal. This was his reply: "Up until I received your letter I simply felt that I made a right request to donate my organs, and therefore it would not only be granted but expedited with relative ease. . . . Your letter served once again to reveal my ignorance. . . . My decision to donate is simply motivated out of a Christian concern for my fellow man. I was not even aware of your existence, let alone of your protracted battle in what's essentially not only a right cause, but one that may save a number of lives."

I immediately pressed Montana authorities to honor King's request. I wrote to them that general anesthesia is the optimal way to go about it and that lethal injection would impair most organs for transplant purposes. The kidneys could be used, but only if removed *immediately* after pronouncement of death—which would mean performing the operation right there in the execution chamber. The time consumed in certifying the victim's death would be critical. With each passing minute the heart's nervelike conduction system deteriorates, and as a transplantable organ it rapidly becomes unsalvageable. And too much time would be needed for the technically more difficult removal of the liver, not to mention the more fragile lungs.

The Corrections Department of the State of Montana answered with the patently evasive explanation that King's request had been referred to the official regional organ procurement agency. Once again drawing upon my experience with such officials, I shot back that without a doubt the agency would ignore the request, and that therefore I myself must be allowed to at least take King's kidneys.

There was little doubt that my dogged and (for the corrections officials) very unwelcome persistence caused a good deal of consternation. My suspicion was confirmed when the execution date was postponed for two months. I knew that things were really buzzing when a reporter acquainted with most of Montana's death row inmates called me for details of what I had in mind.

And it looked as though another of my suspicions was about to be confirmed; namely, that authorities, trapped between what they habitually are wont to do and what they instinctively know is right, would consider dodging the dilemma by granting clemency. I told this to King when (at his request) I telephoned him before his clemency hearing scheduled for mid-January 1989. He tended to agree with my guess that clemency would be granted, as indeed it was. But his attorney denied that it was a move merely to dodge the issue.

I cannot escape the notion that as my campaign gains momentum and spawns an epidemic of such dilemmas, eventually a hopelessly ambivalent and philosophically bankrupt society will escape from its self-imposed impasse by doing away with capital punishment—this time for good. Opponents of the death penalty may therefore unwittingly be obstructing their own cause by remaining silent on, or by actively resisting, the only recent development that is new and powerful enough to help them succeed.

Jonathan Wayne Nobles also gave me his support from death row in Huntsville, Texas. He wrote that "organ donation is something that I have been trying to accomplish from the day I was sentenced to death—October 1987. I have written letter after letter to the A.M.A., the A.C.L.U., Amnesty Int. and many other org. But as yet not one of my letters has been answered." Nobles also stretched out his appeals, he admitted, in order to gain time "to be allowed to die and at the same time give life."

Similar sentiments came from Robert Birch* on death row in Huntingdon, Pennsylvania. His letter began: "First, let me state that I am receptive to the idea of donating my organs; and, in fact, I looked into the possibilities several years ago, only to learn (from the prison doctor) that organ donation is not feasible after electrocution."

Birch mentioned that the Pennsylvania legislature was debating the issue of lethal injection, which he hoped would be legalized (and it was legalized in 1990). Furthermore, he felt that in time the matter would be academic because the state supreme court was considering a serious challenge to the death penalty.

Of special interest is Birch's analysis of the potentially disadvantageous link between organ procurement and lethal injection: "Most legislators are not sympathetic to us," he complained, "and would tend to balk at *any* request from us that would make the sentence 'easier,' no matter what the benefit would be . . . (and lethal injection is viewed as easier than frying)."

Birch's second letter, in January 1989, conveyed the news that lethal injection had not been adopted and that Pennsylvania's death penalty statute had been upheld. He feared that an execution would soon take place, and solemnly concluded that "if it comes to such a point in my case, I will start my own litigation . . . in an attempt to assert my right to donate my organs."

Especially relevant encouragement came in a letter dated 10 March 1989 from Joseph Roger O'Dell, III, who was condemned to die in the electric chair at Boydton, Virginia. In part he said: "I fully see what you are trying to do, and I think that you are misunderstood by many. Your intentions are not macabre, but rather the most kind and humane that I can think of. . . . If your proposal were looked at intelligently, in the proper perspective, and all facets of your proposal taken as a whole, it could be seen that what you suggest gives HOPE to those that are without it, both to the condemned person, and to the person that will be the recipient of the condemned person's organs."

Why especially relevant? Because with his letter O'Dell had enclosed copies of newspaper articles about the death in another state of his seventeen-year-old stepson from severe injuries sustained in an automobile accident. The youth was declared brain-dead after six days in a coma, and O'Dell's wife gave doctors permission to remove organs for transplantation. How ironic that fate would accord an innocent, young son (left brain-dead from an accident) the dignity and beneficence of death denied to his condemned, contrite, and altruistic stepfather. And what appalling hypocrisy among doctors, who must assume most of the responsibility for that immoral denial.

The most prolific correspondent and consistent collaborator in my campaign is Richard Norman Rojem, Jr., a former Michigan resident now on Oklahoma's death row in McAlester. In his first letter Rojem said that my inquiry came as a pleasant surprise because he is a documented organ donor in both states and had been thinking of contacting medical authorities about the possibility of actually donating. "I don't much care for publicity of any kind," he wrote. "But that doesn't mean that I won't do what has to be done to talk to whoever you send—what we want to do here is bigger than the feelings of one man."

Like many others, thirty-two-year-old Rojem is self-taught and fairly astute in criminal law. Consequently he planned carefully for the steps he must take in advancing the campaign. We have coordinated our efforts through telephone calls and many letters. He has sent to prison authorities well-worded statements of his desire to be an organ donor if and when executed. Rojem's activism has brought him into the local limelight, which he dislikes but knows is essential.

In the meantime, *The Detroit News*, Michigan's leading newspaper, became interested in Rojem's involvement because of his Michigan background. It ran a story, based on copies of our correspondence and on special interviews with me and Rojem, about our collaborative effort. The article was published on 30 January 1989 and moved on the wire serving more than ninety Gannett Corporation newspapers, the largest newspaper chain in the world. Newspapers in Oklahoma picked it up and thereby focused interest on Rojem's predicament.

I could see now that my decision to work "from the bottom up" was beginning to pay off. Increasing pressure from death row inmates eventually captured the attention of a couple of organizations dedicated to the abolition of capital punishment, which in turn led to national exposure through an item in *Newsweek*. Suddenly interviewers from radio call-in talk shows began calling me, and I was only too happy to oblige.

And the exposure for Rojem was equally effective. He couldn't believe the sudden change in attitude on the part of authorities in Oklahoma. Until the story broke he had been ignored, and even despised. Suddenly he was the center of attention. His well-conducted letter-writing campaign drew favorable responses from the director of the corrections department, from its medical director, the state's chief medical examiner, and several state legislators; and the latter began serious discussion about pertinent enabling legislation. I followed up with a salvo of complementary letters to clarify technical and medical details and to reinforce Rojem's vigorous challenge.

My participation in a radio telephone talk program in Georgia helped the cause of Mitchell Terry Mincey, whom I had previously contacted by letter on death row in Jackson, Georgia. This twenty-eight-year-old inmate also wanted the state to offer lethal injection instead of electrocution so that he would be able to donate organs. In a short but pithy essay Mincey urged friends and relatives to join in trying to persuade legislators in Atlanta to legitimate the choice.

A local reporter heard me on the radio and prepared an extensive article based on interviews with Mincey, Ronald Spivey (who is also on death row at Jackson, and sympathetic to my cause), several state legislators, and three local doctors.[25] All in all, the published comments tended to be favorable, but guardedly so from the doctors.

After thirty long, disappointing years my lone voice on the outside, amplified by those from death row, finally was loud enough to at least begin to be heard and even heeded.

Here was more proof that the time was ripe.

8

Some "Circus Trick"!

The desk clerk rushed to answer the telephone., "Royal Oak City Hospital, East Surgical Ward. May I help you?"

"This is Warden Jones at the Ohio Penitentiary. I'd like to speak with orderly Harry Eloyan, please. It's quite urgent."

"One moment." Cupping her hand over the mouthpiece, the clerk sent the nurses' aide to tell Harry to take the call in the orderly room. It was 2:00 A.M. when the aide interrupted Harry's reading: "You have a long distance call from Ohio!"

"Ohio?" From who?" he asked rhetorically as he lifted the receiver to his ear. "Hello, this is Harry Eloyan."

"Mr. Eloyan, I'm Warden Jones at the Ohio Penitentiary in Columbus. I'm calling at the suggestion of our medical director, Dr. Ronald Senteau. He says that you are the right man to help us out on an important project. I can't give details over the phone, but you'll see what I mean when you get here. Can you make it?"

"I'm ready to help Dr. Senteau any time," the puzzled orderly replied, trying to regain composure after this mild shock.

"I realize," the warden continued, "how inconvenient it will be for you to drive down from Michigan. Could you be here by noon, or one o'clock at the latest?"

"Inconvenience is putting it mildly," Eloyan mused to himself. He was on the midnight shift that week and wouldn't be free until 7:00 A.M. "It'll be tight, but I think I can get a friend to cover for me so that I can leave right away." He had no doubt that his counterpart on the West Ward would do it, especially on that relatively quiet night. It was customary for them to cooperate like that.

"By the way, we'll need a good X-ray technician, too," the warden added. "Can you bring one along? Dr. Senteau has arranged for all the necessary equipment to be available for you."

"No problem. I have a couple of good friends in the Radiology Department. I'm sure I can talk one of them into coming along." Harry had Joyce Nagel in mind because she was competent, friendly, cooperative to the point of self-sacrifice, and had the next two days off.

"Good! Then we'll expect you around noon. Goodbye, and thank you."

Eloyan's tranquil night of reading now turned hectic. He rushed to the West Ward orderly room to arrange for his drowsy friend to cover his absence. After informing the head nurse on his own ward of the change, he returned to his quarters for a quick shave and to change into street clothes. Grabbing his bagged lunch, he bounded down two flights of stairs to the basement X-ray department to check the duty roster. Yes, Joyce was free for the next two days.

It was 2:20 A.M. when Harry telephoned. "Joyce," he almost shouted, "something very important has come up, and I need your help."

"At this time of night?" she drawled half asleep and with a touch of reproach.

"I can't give you details yet, but it's urgent. Can you leave right away with me for Columbus, Ohio?"

Now fully awake and titillated by a mixture of curiosity and the promise of unexpected adventure, Joyce agreed to be ready in half an hour.

"Great! I'll pick you up at three o'clock. Grab something for breakfast." Harry hung up excitedly and dashed out to the partly deserted parking lot streaked with the gloomy shadows of summertime moonlight. He literally sprang into his brand new Model A Ford and sped off through quiet streets to the other side of town where, at 2:55 A.M., he was knocking on Joyce's door. She was ready.

As he escorted her to his idling car, both were tacitly asking themselves what this was all about.

They headed south on U.S. 24 with Harry at the wheel. Long periods of reflective silence were punctuated by Harry's reminiscences about having served as a medical corpsman under Dr. Senteau's command during the Great War, about how skillful and dedicated the doctor was, and about their close and enduring friendship. They hadn't seen each other for several years now; but if Dr. Senteau turns to Harry for help, then it *has* to be important—and especially for the warden to call at such an ungodly hour.

Joyce understood with frequent nods. Her excitement permitted only brief lapses into light sleep as the sun broke over the horizon to their left.

It turned out to be a gorgeous day. A lovely, cool, and sunny summer day. Nearing Columbus they seemed to be racing fluffy cumulus clouds dotting the light blue sky and wafting on a gentle northwesterly breeze. The splendid weather seemed to reflect the upbeat mood of the entire nation. It was 1929, a year that promised to fulfill those sanguine hopes we all shout on New Year's Eve. But not quite for everyone on this day.

Harry had made good time. At 12:08 P.M. he and Joyce entered Warden Jones's office. After the necessary introductions they settled into comfortable chairs to await Dr. Senteau, whom the warden summoned immediately with a phone call to the infirmary.

Every meeting between Harry and the doctor invariably demonstrated their deep bonds of friendship and mutual respect. As Dr.

Senteau entered, Harry leaped to his feet for a hearty handshake, but was mischievously thwarted when the doctor clasped Harry in a tight embrace of nostalgia accented with joyous laughter and pats on the back. Then they took their seats and got down to business. Time was short.

"I'm sure you both want to know what this is all about," the warden began, alternating his gaze between the two guests. "I'm also sure that you realize how important a matter it must be for me to cause you both so much bother."

Harry and Joyce nodded assent almost involuntarily with their interest aroused to fever pitch. Glancing aside quickly, Harry noticed Dr. Senteau staring directly at him, a wry smile indenting his cheeks. He knew the doctor well and surmised that the smile could signify something only beneficent: throughout their long and intimate association that remarkable doctor had never displayed a jot of malice toward anybody. Whatever was in store, it had to be good.

The warden again drew Harry's attention: "You know that we have capital punishment in Ohio."

Harry nodded at the implied question. "What's that got to do with me?" he thought to himself.

Joyce now began to wonder what Harry had talked her into, as she eyed him nervously.

"Well," Warden Jones continued, "just last month we electrocuted two men and a woman. Another man is scheduled for two o'clock this afternoon, and I . . ."

Dr. Senteau was keenly aware of the pair's mounting anxiety and interrupted the warden. "Maybe it had better come from me," he suggested. "Listen, Harry. Remember those long discussions we used to have in the field hospital at Cambrai near the end of the war?"

Harry nodded hesitantly, still puzzled.

"*You* know," the doctor prompted, "about all that physiological research you were so fascinated with."

Harry's eyes brightened. "I sure do! Boy, what crazy ideas I had about becoming a doctor and some day having the chance to do that kind of research. Pretty naive and stupid, now that I think back on it."

"Don't be so hard on yourself," the doctor chided. "It's not your fault that you couldn't afford to go to college. Besides, I'm a better judge of your talents than you are, and that's why you're here."

"For what?" Harry inquired impatiently. "What can I do that's so special, that someone here in Columbus can't do?"

"Maybe someone here can," retorted Dr. Senteau, "but we don't have time to find out. I *know* you can do it, and right now that's all that counts. Remember those articles and pictures you showed me years ago—about research in France on heart and lung physiology?"

At that instant it began to dawn on Harry what the doctor had in mind. He recalled those French medical publications from the previous century describing experiments dealing with the insertion of tubes into the veins and hearts of animals. Especially vivid was his recollection of a picture showing a man standing by a horse and holding a tube as thick as a hose which had been put through the animal's jugular vein into the heart. Was that what Dr. Senteau was going to try on the condemned man?

"And," the doctor continued, "your suggestion that the same experiment should be tried on a human, and your insistence on how safe it had to be?"

"I sure do," blurted Harry. "And you had to bring me to my senses. In fact, Dr. Senteau, you couldn't see how it could possibly be tried on a human for the first time. But we both agreed that repeating animal experiments would not accomplish much."

"Right!" the doctor exclaimed. "But something new has come up to change things. You may not have heard that the death penalty law in Ohio has been amended to add a choice for condemned criminals."

Warden Jones took advantage of a slight pause. "Correct. We're the first state to offer a choice between the electric chair and anesthesia."

"Not anesthesia alone," the doctor added, "but only if the condemned man will permit medical experiments while he's under. And he'll never wake up."

Harry let out a little whistle, and Joyce was transfixed with astonishment.

Without hesitation the warden continued: "The man who will die at two o'clock is a twenty-five-year-old murderer. And he seems to be genuinely sorry for his crime. He's the first one to decide for anesthesia. We asked him several months ago, and he had until last week to decide. He chose anesthesia right away, without flinching, and hasn't wavered since."

"And he doesn't care at all what experiment is to be done on him, just as long as he doesn't wake up," Dr. Senteau added. "We've wracked our brains trying to figure exactly what is to be tried on him and who is to do it. Every doctor we contacted refused to even consider taking part. Finally, just last night I hit upon the perfect experiment to try."

"Must be the one we've been talking about," interjected Harry. "I take it that Joyce and I are going to help Dr. Senteau do it on the condemned man."

"No, not exactly," countered the doctor.

Harry's zeal faltered. "Why not?" he thought to himself. But his saddened demeanor was quickly dissipated by the doctor's explanation.

"You are going to do it all, Harry—and alone, too!" Senteau meticulously emphasized every word. "If I were going to carry out the experiment myself, I could get all the help I needed right here. Why would I have to bother you in Michigan?"

"But why me instead of you, Dr. Senteau?"

"It's a touchy problem for me, Harry. You see, the state has made it legal to do experiments on willing condemned men, but the medical profession has declared that to be unethical. Personally I can't risk being censured or jeopardizing the standing of the Corrections Department's medical service in the eyes of the profession."

Harry understood the doctor's predicament and nodded agreement.

"No doctor in Ohio dares participate for that reason, Harry. In fact, not many of them even talk about it. But I recalled your enthusiasm over those French experiments, and if anyone from another state has to do it, I knew that you were the man to contact."

"But," Harry queried, "will they let me do it? After all, I'm not a doctor, or even a research assistant."

"It'll be okay," the doctor said assuringly. "The law was worded in accordance with a unique code of ethics recently published in Europe to cover this kind of situation. And the code stipulates that *something* of value must be gotten, even if it takes an interested and able layman to do the research.[4] You fit the bill, Harry."

Now emotionally overwrought, the orderly could barely speak. He began slowly: "Dr. Senteau—you want me to attempt on this condemned man what we talked about at Cambrai?"

"Definitely! I'll be there to watch and to give you moral and technical support if you need it. But I cannot actively take part."

Harry's mind was at full speed. "We'll need a ureteral catheter and a . . ."

The doctor stopped him short. "Don't worry. Everything you need is already there." Turning to Joyce, he continued: "Miss Nagel, we have a portable X-ray machine for you. Also, you might have to help Harry with the anesthesia."

She nodded silently, apprehensive over the looming challenge, especially because she had no experience with general anesthesia.

Presciently, Dr. Senteau continued: "It won't be too difficult. Harry had plenty of experience during the war, and he'll show you how you can help. Just watch him closely."

The warden glanced at his pocket watch. "It's one ten. Time for a quick snack if you're hungry. Dr. Senteau will show you to the staff lounge. We'll meet here in my office at one thirty, and I'll escort you to the execution chamber."

Dr. Senteau had already eaten lunch and began filling in details while Joyce and Harry washed down a sandwich with a cup or two of coffee. "You should know that this is no ordinary execution chamber. You won't see an electric chair. The warden had an old utility room emptied of everything but a few tables and a dozen chairs. In case you need it, there's a sink with running water in one corner. The outside wall has two large barred windows. The condemned man will be lying on a big table in the center of the room. Harry, you and Joyce can use the two smaller tables. One of them has all the material you'll need for the experiment. Let me know if anything is missing when you check things over. The lighting is bad, so the warden had a couple of floor model goose-neck lamps brought in."

Harry's attention was strained as he simultaneously ruminated on the procedure he was to follow in carrying out the experiment. It was simple enough, and he could recall every detail vividly.

Turning directly toward Joyce, the doctor continued: "A portable X-ray machine and two lead aprons were borrowed from the University Hospital. I'm sure you're familiar with this model, Joyce." She smiled and nodded.

"Things should go smoothly, Harry. I gave the condemned man pentobarbital a little while ago; he wanted something to calm him down. I shouldn't be criticized for that. After all, it's merely treating a patient and has nothing to do with executing someone." The doctor then looked at his pocket watch." My gosh, it's almost 1:30. Let's go!"

The three met the warden leaving his office. "Great timing," he said anxiously. "So far everything is right on schedule."

They passed two door guards and entered a large, newly painted, rectangular room with a ceiling at least ten feet high. The smoothly plastered walls were ivory colored, the floor a dark beige. In the center a supine man covered with a white sheet lay on a large wooden table. His head rested comfortably on a small white pillow, immobile, eyes fixed blankly on the ivory ceiling. Behind his head were a chair and a small table, on which sat three cans of ether and three gauze masks. At the man's feet and to his left was a similar small table bearing the paraphernalia Harry needed. On the right was the X-ray machine. The two lead aprons were slung over a chair against the outside wall. Along that wall and the opposite inside wall was a single row of plain chairs. All but two were occupied by spectators, most of whom were newspaper reporters; but included were a minister, a priest, a judge, a criminologist, the convict's attorney—and strangely, a man in a guard's uniform.

Soft murmuring stopped abruptly as the warden began to introduce his three companions. He also pointed out the open windows and repeated his warning that there was to be absolutely no smoking or lighted flame of any kind in the room. He and Dr. Senteau then took their seats along the outside wall near the door. A specially installed telephone was on the floor at the warden's feet.

Dr. Senteau looked at the clock on the opposite wall and motioned to Harry and Joyce who were still standing just inside the doorway. Joyce went to the X-ray machine to make sure that everything was in order. Four large film cassettes were on the chair beneath the lead aprons.

Harry proceeded to the small table behind the convict's head. Everything seemed to be there: A thin, sterile ureteral catheter; a large, sterile aneurysm needle; a large syringe filled with 50 ccs of concentrated potassium chloride solution to which a 20-gauge needle was attached; a small bottle of tincture of iodine; a sterile scalpel and blade; a pile of sterile 4-by-4-inch gauze pads; a roll of white adhesive tape; and two pairs of sterile rubber gloves.

Harry swung the small table to the convict's shoulder, reached under the sheet and pulled the man's left arm straight out to rest on the table, perpendicular to the trunk of his body. Harry then stood still.

An eerie silence ensued as everybody's eyes focused on the wall clock. At two minutes to two the phone rang, and the message came down from the governor's office. Reprieve denied. Dr. Senteau signaled with a wave of his hand. Harry opened a can of ether, picked up a gauze mask, and sat down behind the convict's head.

At exactly 2:00 P.M. Harry placed the mask over the convict's nose and mouth and soaked it with ether. He kept dripping ether onto the mask as the convict's breathing became stertorous* and his body reacted with mild agitation. Soon the convict was totally unconscious and breathing uniformly. It was time to begin the experiment.

Joyce was solidifying Harry's prior briefing on ether anesthesia by watching him closely. She felt confident in taking over and freeing him to don a pair of rubber gloves. Using gauze dipped in iodine Harry swabbed the inner surface of the convict's left elbow. After nicking the skin with a scalpel blade, Harry punctured the vein with

---

*Loud and harsh sounding.

the aneurysm needle, into which he immediately inserted the tip of the ureteral catheter. Packing the area with gauze, he taped the needle in place and began slowly pushing the catheter up the vein in the convict's left arm. Harry stopped when the two-foot mark on the catheter reached the aneurysm needle. According to prior external measurements, the inserted end of the catheter must have entered the right ventricle of the heart.

Harry secured the catheter on the forearm with adhesive tape and asked Joyce to interrupt the ether drip in order to take X-rays. Joyce donned a lead apron, positioned the machine to the right of the convict, slipped a film cassette under his chest, and aimed the X-ray beam directly down on it for a front-to-back shot.

Harry then put down the can of ether, put on the other apron, turned the inmate onto his right side, and held him there for two lateral films. The convict was again laid supine with the catheter still in place. Harry felt the pulse; it was regular and strong. There was no sign of distress.

Joyce doffed her apron, turned off the machine, and took all four cassettes to the infirmary for developing. Harry resumed the ether drip. He looked at the clock to his left; it was fifteen after two. What now? They had neglected to tell him how this ceremony was to end. He threw a troubled glance at Dr. Senteau who already had signaled one of the spectators.

Harry was surprised to see the man in the guard's uniform rise and approach him. He leaned over and whispered to Harry: "I'm the executioner. I'm to give him an injection to finish it."

Somewhat taken aback, Harry pointed out the syringe filled with a lethal dose of potassium chloride and instructed the man to inject it rapidly by piercing the catheter near its entrance into the vein. Harry stopped the ether drip and put the gauze mask aside to watch. The injection was done adeptly. For several seconds the unconscious subject gurgled softly, and his breathing became light and irregular. He then turned ashen, his mouth sagged wider, and he lay perfectly still.

Dr. Senteau arose, approached the lifeless form with a stethoscope in his hand, and listened for heart sounds. Nothing. It was 2:19 P.M.

Once again, justice had been served. But this time, for the first time, all of humankind had also been served.

So far, this story is partly fiction. Why? To find out, you'll have to take a mental trip four thousand miles east of Columbus, to a suburban hospital in Berlin, Germany.[16] It is shortly after noon of an early summer day in 1929. Here we meet twenty-five-year-old Dr. Werner Forssmann. The aspiring surgeon finally succeeded in talking a sympathetic operating room nurse into helping him with an experiment that had been strictly forbidden by the chief of his department. He was not to try it on anyone, including himself.

Dr. Forssmann was fascinated by reports published in the nineteenth century by French researchers who had been studying the cardiopulmonary physiology in animals by means of transvenous catheters into the heart. The picture of the horse with the hoselike tube in its vein was indelibly burned into Dr. Forssmann's memory. He was convinced that the procedure would be innocuous for humans, and extremely valuable for both drug therapy and for more accurate diagnosis. He was determined to prove it and thereby break a taboo that placed heart surgery beyond the realm of possibility.

Dr. Forssmann had a friendly and sympathetic chief of surgery who agreed with his young protege's ideas and aims, but who could not risk his professional reputation and position by permitting such an outlandish experiment. Nevertheless, despite his promise to the contrary, the irascible young doctor planned to go ahead and do it on himself. With carefully calculated attention and flattery over several weeks, Dr. Forssmann eventually won the support of the head nurse and thereby guaranteed access to the necessary instruments. He did this by implying that the experiment would be performed on her, with the assurance that there was absolutely no danger.

The lull of the customary noontime break offered the best time to try it. The nurse lay on a table in a small cubicle while Dr. Forssmann pretended to work on her arm. With deliberate slowness he swabbed her elbow area with iodine solution and then, out of sight behind her head, quickly set to work on his own vein. Before she caught on to his ruse, Dr. Forssmann had swabbed his elbow, nicked the locally anesthetized skin, pierced his vein, and inserted the catheter into it up to his shoulder region.

The nurse was only momentarily peeved at having been duped, and cooperated by going to the X-ray department to alert the technician as Dr. Forssmann had asked. He then advanced the catheter to the two-foot mark, got up, and walked to the X-ray room where everything was ready for fluoroscopy and filming.

At Dr. Forssmann's request the technician had set up a mirror so that he could see the screen. The tip of the catheter was indeed in the right ventricle. Postero-anterior and lateral films were taken to document results.

Word of the experiment spread rapidly throughout the hospital. A colleague burst into the room and shouted, "Are you crazy?" He even tried to yank the catheter out before X-rays were taken, but Dr. Forssmann blocked the attempt. On learning of the extraordinary event, the chief surgeon was upset that Dr. Forssmann had broken his promise. But he was relieved at the outcome and cognizant of its importance. He urged Dr. Forssmann to write an article without delay and even helped compose it. The landmark report was published in an authoritative German medical journal about six months later.

In the meantime, knowing that Dr. Forssmann hoped for a career in research, the chief helped him secure a nonpaid position under the world-famous, highly skilled, and strong-willed surgeon Ferdinand Sauerbruch at Germany's most prestigious hospital in Berlin. Unhappily, Dr. Forssmann was assigned to menial tasks and felt smothered by an atmosphere, quite like that in many of our academic institutions today, where "radical" independent thought was considered to be deadly poison. The full force of the oppressive mentality hit Dr. Forssmann immediately after his article appeared in print. Sensational reports in the evening newspapers didn't help his situation. Medical colleagues ignored or denounced the experiment, some brazenly claiming priority of discovery, and a few even accusing him of outright plagiarism.

The really crushing blow was Dr. Sauerbruch's inevitable reaction: that what Dr. Forssmann did might be okay "in a circus . . . but never in a respectable German university!" Dr. Sauerbruch ended a tirade by screaming, "Get out! Leave my department immediately!"[16] Dr. Forssmann felt relieved—just as I did in 1958 when asked to leave the university if I persisted in my campaign.

Over the next few years other investigators, especially Drs. Andrè Cournand and Dickinson Richards, Jr., in the United States, made extensive use of the procedure to vindicate Dr. Forssmann's prophecy that it would prove valuable for therapy and diagnosis, and would expand the horizon of surgery into formerly untouchable areas.

What makes this story so powerful is the fact that a quarter of a century later—after having been scorned, insulted, and vilified by arrogant and pathetically short-sighted colleagues—Dr. Forssmann shared the 1956 Nobel prize for medicine as a well-deserved and unduly belated acknowledgment of his now famous "circus trick"!

Many obvious and irrefutable conclusions can be drawn from all this:

1. Dr. Forssmann was compelled to take an unnecessary risk in 1929 by an irrational attitude on the part of the medical profession and the society it advises. He, or any one of the millions of doctors around the world, could have done it very quickly and easily on a willing condemned criminal in any civilized nation using the death penalty (and use of the penalty was rampant back then). The risk for Dr. Forssmann was magnified because, in contrast to a condemned subject, he was not under general anesthesia. Of course, that might have been one of the reasons for considering his feat to have been of exceptional distinction. In the case of an anesthetized human being who, by law, must be destroyed, there could be absolutely no risk, *no matter what happens!*

2. Almost the same Nobel prize-winning experiment could have been done at any time during the previous century, even by those French physiologists if they had clamored for the condemned's choice of death under some form of anesthesia instead of by the guillotine. I say "almost" because Dr. Forssmann was fully conscious and could

know of any subjective complications, while an anesthetized subject could not. However, once proved to be absolutely and objectively safe under anesthesia, there is little doubt that clinical trials on awake individuals would have followed in short order. One can only guess (and lament) how much faster our current medical marvels would have been achieved and how many tragically premature deaths that alternate course of events could have averted.

3. A series of replicating experiments is not a prerequisite for obtaining valuable and useful results. A single probe could do it, provided that the researcher is bright, inquisitive, highly imaginative, honest, and "gutsy." We all know how rare that combination is, especially in ivory-tower Academe where "dangerous," taboo-smashing intelligence is systematically rooted out and eliminated. Dr. Forssmann can attest to that.

4. No serious experiment on an anesthetized condemned person can be too "silly" or "impractical." What may strike superannuated minds as being a mere "circus trick" today may be the Nobel prizewinner in a philosophically more mature and technologically more advanced society tomorrow. At the very least, no willing condemned man or woman should be put to death without being anesthetized so that the lethal dose of some new or obscure drug or chemical may be determined under those conditions.

5. Doctors or any other professional personnel are not necessary to achieve good results. If they are willing to take part, then paraprofessionals or even qualified lay individuals should be given the opportunity to try—and that is what really counts—to extract something of value from an otherwise totally nihilistic act. Almost any doctor, medical corpsman, technologist, or nurse could have accomplished Dr. Forssmann's feat on an anesthetized convict. That is not to denigrate his epochal achievement, the greatness of which derives not from theoretical or technical complexity, but from the immense amount of courage, strength of character, and will it took to overcome society's formidable and purely arbitrary obstacles. Removal of those obstacles,

which is what I am trying to coax society to do, would have made Dr. Forssmann's goal simple.

6. Valuable experiments need not be gruesome or mutilating. Indeed, Dr. Forssmann's caused no discomfort at all. And neither should the minimal effort already mentioned: that of merely determining an unknown lethal dose.

7. The investigator, whether doctor or layman, could never, with rational justification, be considered an executioner when conducting experiments in the conventional way on such condemned subjects. After all, as a rule the longer a subject lives, the more one can learn. The primary, in fact, the only, aim is to probe and to discover, not to kill. If the subject dies in the process, it would be accidental and no more intentional killing than would be the case with inadvertent death during routine curative surgery in hospitals. And, as in the above dramatized story, if the anesthetized subject were to survive the experiment, then the ultimately lethal action would be the responsibility of a duly authorized lay executioner.

8. Finally, and of easily overlooked importance, execution through anesthetic experimentation would offer a unique advantage which is absolutely unthinkable with any other mode of execution: hitherto impossible "thirteenth" and "fourteenth hour" chances for reprieve. Just imagine that somehow evidence were to be discovered to exonerate the condemned man in the fictionalized version and reported to the governor's office before 2:15 P.M. The falsely condemned subject of the experiment could have been revived intact (and probably in better condition than most postoperative patients in our hospitals) and freed to live a normal life. Depending upon the type of experiment, the period of resuscitability could conceivably extend for several hours, perhaps even a day.

One cannot help but wonder if some unlucky, innocent soul among the 5,000 or so criminals executed in the United States since 1900 would not have escaped an ugly and totally unjust fate if allowed to submit to anesthesia and one of those outlandish "circus tricks."

9

The Hypocritic Oafs

I was invited in 1960 to appear before the Joint Legislative Committee on Capital Punishment in Columbus, Ohio. Fortunately, my booklet entitled "Medical Research and the Death Penalty," published earlier that year, was available to strengthen my presentation at the committee hearing. Determined to overcome the stonewalling by the medical press, I hoped that the booklet would bring my proposal to the attention not only of the medical community but the public at large—and thereby stimulate discussion. Despite meager promotion and distribution, the booklet did receive reviews in several national and state medical journals. They ranged from noncommittal to enthusiastic acclaim; but most important, not one denounced the booklet or its content.

At the prior request of the committee chairman, I sent copies to a dozen or more famous researchers for their opinions regarding the idea's potential *medical* value only. A few of them simply rejected my proposal out of hand because they were opposed to capital punishment. One such critic was a Nobel laureate whose prize-winning work could have been done earlier, easier, cheaper, and more safely under the conditions of my proposal.

Other respondents merely acknowledged receipt of the booklet or gave tangential approval of my proposal. Only four replies were honestly forthright. In two of them another Nobel laureate and a world-famous pioneer in heart surgery admitted the soundness of my proposal, but volunteered that open endorsement of it would probably cost them their professorships at their respective universities. The only unconditional support was given by a preeminent Boston pathologist, Dr. Arthur Purdy Stout, and noted neurophysiologist, Dr. Ralph Gerard of Ann Arbor, Michigan (both of whom are now deceased).

I arrived in Columbus several hours before the committee meeting and decided to find out what one or two staff doctors at the Ohio State University Hospital thought of my proposal. In the hallway of the Department of Surgery I chanced upon an associate professor who expressed willingness to answer a question I wanted to put to him. I explained my proposal and my reason for soliciting his opinion. On learning what it was about, his friendliness suddenly disappeared as he rejected the concept unequivocally.

Then I asked: "If *you* were on death row and chose not to die under anesthesia and experimentation, would you at least prefer to have had the choice to refuse and be electrocuted, or instead be forced to die in the electric chair without having a choice?" I knew he would try to justify his stance with the outlandish decision of allowing no choice whatsoever; and he did just that, and angrily, too. Accustomed to, and exasperated by, such professional evasiveness, I departed with a less than amiable farewell, saving the bulk of my passion for the crucial hearing at the capitol.

Combined with the few unconditional medical endorsements I had received, my booklet and oral arguments were enough to convince the committee members of the merit of my endeavor. But capital punishment was waning in the United States, and this made further vigorous campaigning on my part almost meaningless. However, the proposal was never out of my mind. Death rows were not abolished or vacated during the moratorium, and I still pursued the idea in a low-key way whenever a likely opportunity arose. For example, when condemned inmates were the subject of news items, I wrote to them. And if I was traveling near a major prison, I tried to get permission to interview men on death row—but I never succeeded.

Throughout the decade and a half from 1960 to the mid-1970s, during which no executions were carried out in the United States, I continued to solicit favorable opinions from well-known doctors. However, as before, almost all of them either ignored my inquiry or rejected the idea solely on the (irrelevant) basis of their personal dislike of the death penalty.

But the late Professor Hans Selye of Montreal was different. Like Drs. Stout and Gerard more than ten years earlier, he agreed that the concept did indeed have medical value, provided the condemned had a free choice in the matter and that uninterrupted anesthesia would be carefully monitored.

It was now time to get the campaign off the back burner. In the latter half of the 1970s, executions in the United States were once again on the upswing. The legislative debate over switching to lethal injection in Oklahoma, Texas, Idaho, and New Mexico was full of emotion and even medical nonsense. The issue was raised initially in Oklahoma for humanitarian as well as for economic reasons. There wasn't much doubt that the new method would ease suffering and at the same time substantially reduce costs. Oklahoma's electric chair had been mothballed since 1966, and refurbishing it would have cost more than sixty thousand dollars. Switching to lethal gas and building a chamber for it would have cost four times as much. On the other hand, a single execution by lethal drug injection could be accomplished for a paltry ten to fifteen dollars.[17]

There was no room for argument or emotional doubletalk about the economic advantages. But the death penalty's broad philosophical implications made any innovation, no matter how advantageous, vulnerable to attack by the antagonistic members of the medical hierarchy who oppose capital punishment.

One of their first moves is to label any doctor unethical who would either insert the needle into a condemned man's vein or actually do the injecting to cause death. They claim that it violates the so-called Hippocractic Oath. I say "so-called," because the oath's origin and content are not clearly understood and its real meaning is often misconstrued. But more will be said about that in chapter 11.

Another of their "arguments" is that medicine is diminished to the extent that it accedes to the use of its lifesaving tools in attempts to civilize the death penalty. They go so far as to claim it unethical for any doctor to prescribe or otherwise help make available the drugs used. This is carried to the extreme of positing no moral difference between a doctor merely supplying the drugs for the injection and a doctor who actually injects for the purpose of killing.

Despite desperate ploys by the opposition, Oklahoma became the first state to adopt lethal injection in May 1977. Seven years later I contacted the state senator who had sponsored the legislation, asking what he thought of my proposal. The senator was surprised to learn that I had advocated the choice of lethal injection almost two decades earlier. He praised as "most refreshing" the "intellectual honesty" of my current position, and denounced as "abhorrent" the hypocrisy of the medical testimony at his legislative sessions.

Three other states soon followed Oklahoma's lead. The first was Texas, where legislators correctly decided that the electric chair was too much like a medieval torture device; later Idaho and New Mexico followed suit.

But these successes didn't stop the wrangling. Spokespersons for organized medicine kept fueling the flames of controversy with complaints that the use of drugs for judicial killing merely added respectable veneer to an act of deliberate and dehumanizing barbarism. Nevertheless many doctors experienced frustrating levels of personal ambivalence. Under relentless pressure the Oklahoma legislature, in the end, exempted doctors from the duty of performing the injections, and the Oklahoma Medical Association then took a neutral position with regard to the new method of execution.

The medical director of the state's Corrections Department, Dr.

Armond Start, foresaw no ethical problem for any doctor who ordered the drugs which were to be used, or who simply inspected the arrangement of tubes and syringes to assure proper flow of the lethal mixture. He said: "I am going to order these drugs. How they're used is none of my business. Our medical people are not going to be involved except to see that the highest standards of medicine are followed."[17]

On the other hand, for Dr. Charles Steuart, Medical Director of Idaho's prison system, any doctor who went beyond merely pronouncing death would be acting unethically. His emotionalism even led him to foresee medical involvement culminating in doctors torturing prisoners and in repeating the Nazi crimes.[17]

The negative overtones extended to Florida where pressure from Dr. Richard Hodes helped defeat a plan to substitute lethal injection for the electric chair. Wielding the impressive credentials of medical doctor, anesthesiologist, president of the Florida State Medical Association, and state legislative representative, Hodes was "very uncomfortable with a technique that is used routinely for healing purposes also used to destroy human life." He warned that lethal injection would probably take five to ten minutes to kill; and if done incompetently, the effect of the thiopental might wear off and let the unconscious condemned inmate suffocate as a result of total muscle paralysis.[17]

His preference for electrocution was backed by Dr. Ronald Wright, Chief Medical Examiner of Dade County and an expert on electrocution. According to Wright, "It takes less than a minute. . . . The prisoner feels no pain because, at least *in theory* (italics added), the electrical impulses travel to the brain's pain receptors and short-circuit them before the sensation of electricity has had time to reach those same receptors via the nerves. The brutality of electrocution is inflicted on the witnesses and on the prisoner's unfeeling body."[18]

The reader is probably wondering—with me—how Wright could be so confident that theory corresponds exactly with what really happens in the victim's mind and body. His tenuous conclusion reiterates that of a group of doctors who witnessed the first four executions using electricity in New York a century earlier: "They were most satisfactory, . . . death was instantaneous and painless in each instance.

. . . This was unquestionably a method superior to any yet devised for the purpose."[18]

As was mentioned in chapter 4, the first execution by lethal injection took place in Texas on 7 December 1982. It was ineptly done by three nonmedical prison employees. The prison doctor witnessed it and was criticized by medical colleagues for having examined the condemned man's badly scarred veins to help those who were to do the injecting, and for saying that he himself could have performed it easier.

That event rekindled the debate. In 1983 Oklahoma's medical director of the Corrections Department, Dr. Start, insisted that doctors should not be executioners, that thousands of people can be trained to do the injecting, and that he personally would not train them— even though he would not brand other doctors as unethical if they did the injecting or training. But Start's underlying ambivalence was exposed by the admission that he or some other doctor should be present to take over in case of difficulty, "to avoid doing harm," as he put it.[19] In that roundabout way he admits the immorality on the part of the medical profession in withholding the *best* means of attaining what society deems to be a legitimate and moral aim.

Oklahoma State Senator Bill Dawson emphasized that point by asking, "If health care providers don't insure the process is done correctly and humanely, who will? Health professionals," he continued, "cannot excuse themselves from the responsibility of executing lethal injection."[19]

Dr. Start responded by citing that part of the Hippocratic Oath which exhorts a doctor to "do no harm." He said, "I, as a physician, cannot be involved with any prisoner in any professional relationship that is not intended to improve or evaluate his physical or mental health."[19]

Come, now, Dr. Start—do you really believe that mental well-being, at least, of a condemned inmate couldn't possibly be improved through the anticipation and experiencing of a painless injection by a skilled doctor, instead of a "painless" death in the electric chair, as theorized by Dr. Wright? And would you have us believe that if *you* were that condemned man, your mental state wouldn't be a bit more troubled in anticipation of a lethal injection by someone other than a skilled doctor?

In 1983 a group of condemned convicts took advantage of the controversy over lethal injection in order to extend their appeals process. Their attorney joined medical authorities in contending that the Federal Drug Administration (FDA) had not yet ruled on the propriety of the alternate, nonmedical use of drugs for lethal injection, and on their safety and effectiveness for that purpose. Ultimately the United States Supreme Court upheld the FDA's sensible position that the decision to use drugs for lethal injection is not within its jurisdiction but is the responsibility of any state which resorts to that method of execution.

The absurdity of the medical profession's stand in this regard is obvious. In October 1983 Dr. Start concluded that lethal injection "is a perversion; an evil use of medicine." But, by strict definition isn't it for *medical* purposes that veterinarians use drugs? In its 1983 publication on euthanasia the Humane Society of the United States recommended as one of the most humane and aesthetically pleasing methods for the mercy killing of animals the injection of pentobarbital by a trained technician. Death is so rapid that the animal collapses before the needle is withdrawn.[20]

Can barbiturates be called—without sounding silly—human medicines only? I have witnessed a veterinary doctor perform euthanasia on a cat that was dying of cancer; he injected pentobarbital, and the animal's reaction was exactly as the Humane Society's publication described. Now, isn't that a legitimate medical use of the drug? And would Dr. Start *dare* call that act a perversion, or the veterinarian's use of the drug an evil? It is this kind of ragged and exceedingly emotional "thinking" that really undermines the medical profession and accounts for much of its lamentable ethical sickness.

Some doctors have the common sense to disagree with Dr. Start and his supporters, and the courage to say so. In 1987 Drs. T. C. Gray and E. S. Sweeney, both of the medical examiner's office in Utah, stated that "to ban all participation of physicians in death sentence cases would raise greater ethical issues than it resolves." Dr. D. L. Wishart, a radiotherapist in Yakima, Washington, agreed that "it is neither possible nor ethically defensible to declare that physicians must refuse to be involved in the *insoluble problem* (italics added) of capital punishment."[21]

Many medical organizations, especially the AMA, are guilty of trying to foster that spurious idealism. According to a resolution passed by the AMA in 1981, "a physician . . . should not be a participant in a legally authorized execution."[19] That admonition might have been innocuous enough before Oklahoma's lethal injection law of 1977, but after that the resolution contradicted a prior tenet in the AMA's own first code of ethics published over a century ago, which obligated ". . . a physician to remember that he is a citizen and *to aid in enforcing laws*" (italics added).[18] And as recently as 1986 the AMA's Council on Ethical and Judicial Affairs proclaimed that "as a citizen and a professional with special training and experience, *the physician has an ethical obligation to assist in the administration of justice*" (italics added).[22] That directly contradicts the AMA's 1981 resolution.

With docile obeisance to AMA policy, in 1983 the American College of Physicians inserted into its revised and ponderous code of ethics—without any discussion or qualification—the same terse injunction that "participation by physicians in the lethal injection of prisoners is unethical."[23]

But the most shocking verbiage came from the American Psychiatric Association, which proclaimed that "killing with lethal injection is wrong; it is *no different* (italics added) than older, more 'barbaric' methods such as drawing and quartering, hanging, and electrocution."[19] Bizarre mentation like that hardly needs comment.

Despite the AMA's official stand against lethal injection, its leaders continued to walk the fence. In 1982 one of its rank and file members wondered if a doctor should be disciplined for unethical conduct if he or she performed lethal injection. The reply from the hierarchy was that even though such behavior "obviously" does not enhance the profession's public image, medical disciplinary action would be unjustified.[24] In other words, a doctor who does the injecting would have committed only a minor, indeed negligible, infringement of ethics at worst. The AMA's ambivalence was showing.

Since 1982, I have contacted twenty-two noted doctors (most of them surgeons) in the United States, Canada, and Europe for their opinions about taking and using organs from the condemned. Only five responded—four Americans and one European. The latter endorsed the idea with the following brief statement: "For various reasons I am personally against capital punishment. If, however, the death penalty is accepted by any society, I would endorse your proposal to permit the removal of organs for transplantation purposes from prisoners condemned to death, who have given assent." This reiterated the outlook of Dr. Jean Hamburger, the noted French transplant surgeon, who, in the 1940s, removed kidneys from criminals immediately after decapitation by guillotine and implanted them into recipients.*

How refreshing! If just a few transplant surgeons in the United States or Canada were as rational, sensible, cooperative, and honest, as a few of their European counterparts, there would be no need for this book.

Among the American respondents was Dr. Charles Bailey, a noted pioneer in heart surgery, now retired, who lent me vigorous support. He wrote to me in September 1986, saying: "I couldn't agree with you more. The need is there (excessively so) and it is wasteful—and even criminal—to permit the healthy organs of these persons who are about to be executed to be denied to the helpless people awaiting transplants."

Contrarily, the other three Americans, including two famous transplant surgeons and an associate dean of a leading medical school (himself active in an organ procurement program), rejected my proposal. In 1987 their letters showed them to be more concerned about what the public's reaction might be than about the proposal's genuine value.

One of them, a noted surgeon, replied by letter in January 1987

---

*Schmeck, *The Semi-artificial Man: A Dawning Revolution in Medicine* (New York: H. M. Walker & Co., 1965), p. 138.

to complain that the philosophic cowardice I had ascribed to another reluctant surgeon "might better be termed discretion." And he added: "The media have taken such an enormous interest in transplantation that it might be prudent not to inflame them with something as titillating as the question of organ donation from condemned criminals."

Two years earlier, in December 1985, the other surgeon admitted having "thought of this possibility in the past" as a partial solution to the shortage of organs. "However," he continued, "we have abstained from supporting such a proposal, feeling that it would shower transplantation with a very bad aura in the mind of the public, and that it might suggest that nefarious motives and secondary gain for others might lead to an increase in capital punishment in general."

Both of these antagonistic surgeons preferred to try to satisfy the demand for organs by stepping up efforts to exploit potential donors among the clinically brain-dead. To date, however, that approach has been a dismal failure.

The associate dean in this group of respondents felt that enough organs would be available if "potential donors are automatically called to the attention of authorized organ procurement organizations." He, too, was worried that "many in the public would view the harvesting of multiple organs from a condemned convict as rather ghoulish and that the negative attitudes engendered by this far outweigh any potential good in terms of the small number of organs made available."

Their objections are dismaying, to say the least, from both a humanitarian and a scientific viewpoint. As discussed in chapter 3, the actual number of organs which might be obtained from death rows is entirely beside the point. My motive for pursuing this campaign is *not* to help alleviate the continuing shortage of organs. Rather, that gain would be just a by-product of my aim to convince a self-centered medical profession and an insouciant society to civilize the way the death penalty is inflicted. As a potential source of organs—limited though it may be—the concept is the most potent "club" available to me with which to "beat" some sense into recalcitrant surgeons, deans, and politicians. As a kind of bait, it embodies the only force or argument they understand and appreciate: the promise of selfish gain in the form of another handy source of organs to help ease the perpetual deficit of donors which causes them so much anguish and a bit of embarrassment. That, together with the added inducement of selfish pecuniary benefit from the increased incidence of highly lucrative surgery thereby engendered, might be enough to lure them to accept this honorable and altruistic concept.

The proclaimed basis of their opposition to my proposal would be deplored by any true scientist. How ludicrous that noted members of a profession, so proud of having achieved a quasi-scientific status, smugly draw conclusions distilled from the "evidence" of their own personal opinions. They reject taking organs from condemned convicts because they "think" they will offend the public and impair their organized procurement programs. Why don't they use some of their immense research resources to gather real, objective evidence from which valid conclusions can be drawn? Isn't that what their vaunted "scientific method" demands?

Despite my meager means, at each step in my campaign I made it a point to gather enough raw data for some kind of reliable indication of the true state of affairs. And my 1984 sample questionnaire, though necessarily limited, revealed that 60 percent to 70 percent of those responding (which included medical personnel) favored my proposal.[3] Such unofficial results may not satisfy surgeons and academicians addicted to double-blind, cross-over, and chi-squared studies; but they constitute tangible, relatively objective evidence, and they *support* my opinion. What *comparable* evidence supports theirs?

Organ procurement agencies also kept prudently silent with regard to my proposal. In January 1983, shortly before a national meeting of a transplantation organization in Washington, D.C., I received a very brief letter from one of its officers, a doctor: "It is clear that many interesting points have been raised in this regard, but I hope you will see it is equally clear that the American Council on Transplantation is not currently prepared to provide a policy statement on this subject. . . . I doubt we will be able to include it in our first program." But the exact reason for the reluctance to provide that policy statement was not given and was anything but clear. And, as

I had expected, the topic was never on the agenda of any subsequent program.

Three years later, in 1986, I had an opportunity to explain details of my proposal to a renowned transplant surgeon during a personal visit to his office in a Detroit hospital. The surgeon agreed that the idea made sense, and he seemed to be supportive of it. Before committing himself in writing, he said that the Organ Procurement Agency of Michigan would have to review the matter. After waiting almost a year for the agency's letter, which arrived in March 1987, I could easily have guessed what the decision would be: "The Board members reviewed the proposal and concluded they did not wish to endorse this controversial proposal." In a moment of carelessness this organization openly admitted having let the dread of controversy override all other considerations.

My criticism here is based on more than personal experience alone. Three death row inmates have written to inform me that their inquiries with regard to possible organ donation when executed were completely ignored by official organ procurement agencies in their respective states.

I know of only one instance in which an agency did agree to collaborate with a surgeon who planned to comply with a prisoner's wish to donate organs at the time of execution. The inmate was a fifty-four-year-old grandmother and murderess condemned to die by lethal injection in North Carolina in November 1984. On her own she had contacted the regional organ procurement agency, which undertook lengthy negotiations to secure the cooperation of legal, judicial, governmental, and corrections authorities. However, because of a lack of organization, multilateral coordination, ethical and technical guidelines, and proper orientation on the part of all parties (all of which this book is aimed at correcting), the heroic attempt by Dr. Jesse H. Meredith to remove the executed woman's kidneys was a dismal failure.[26]

According to Meredith's report, prison officials considered the procedure to be a nuisance and refused to let it be done on site. To complicate matters, the attempt was delayed for twenty minutes after onset of the lethal injection so that her death could be certified beyond doubt. Then the use of all medical facilities in the area was denied. This forced Meredith's team to try to keep the kidneys viable by means of artificial cardiopulmonary resusciation in the ambulance transporting the corpse back to his own hospital 100 miles away at the Bowman Gray School of Medicine! It was futile.

The passive obstructionism from the medical establishment that thwarts the harvesting of organs from death row inmates is especially deplorable, and it doesn't seem to be at all uncommon. For example, in Georgia in February 1989 two men condemned to die in the electric chair requested lethal injection so that their kidneys, at least, could be salvaged. When asked for his opinion, Dr. William S. Hutchings, a family practitioner, agreed that "it would probably be a more humane way to administer capital punishment. But," he added, "if I were sitting on a hospital's board of directors, I would have a very difficult time giving the state permission to use the facility to execute prisoners, even if the organs were going to be removed *and used to save the lives of others*" (italics added).[25]

In the short account of his experience[26] Meredith listed a number of "ifs" that must be resolved for organ procurement from those on death row to be successfully accomplished:

(1) The procurement team must have access to the donor the moment death is declared.

(2) There must be procurement facilities nearby.

(3) Brain death must be the "criterion for execution."

(4) Prison officials have to be sure that removing vital organs is actually fatal.

(5) Vital organs will be removed without chance of resuscitation.

(6) Procurement teams must be assured that they won't be viewed as executioners.[26]

These are "ifs" that my proposal would eradicate. I telephoned him several times in 1987, confident that at last I had found a noted transplant surgeon who would—indeed must—support my campaign without reservation. With some reluctance he agreed that I was doing the right thing; but he failed to give a definitive answer when I asked whether he would be willing to take the kidneys from another convict executed by lethal injection under much more favorable circumstances arranged by me to eliminate every one of his "ifs." I never received written confirmation of his support, which I had requested more than once. And I have not heard from him since those phone calls in 1987.

The equivocation of many doctors is exemplified by several opinions published in connection with the desire of the two Georgia inmates mentioned above. According to a report in a Macon newspaper,[25] Dr. Ellis Evans, a vascular surgeon, and Dr. Carl Lane, a heart surgeon, agreed with Dr. Hutchings that lethal injection would afford a more humane execution. They didn't see "any problem as long as that's what the prisoner wants to do." But all three foresaw enormous ethical and philosophical problems. For instance, Evans was concerned about whether the actual cause of death would be a decision by the judicial system or an act of the medical profession. He was worried about the dilemma for professionals being asked to snuff out the very life they are dedicated to save. He did concede that "the organ would be acceptable, if there weren't any contagious disease. . . . But it would certainly have to be screened quite fully because of the incarceration."

I'll address the ethical and philosophical concerns in chapter 11, but concern about the disease factor is easy to allay and, in fact, should not even have been raised. Evans should know, or at least suspect, that no seriously ill criminal is ever executed in our country. An ailing inmate is always made healthy before being killed, or allowed to die of natural causes if the condition is incurable. Furthermore, convicts usually spend many years on death row where minor ailments are taken care of without delay, and where the opportunity to contract a debilitating, contagious disease is nil. Finally, even a past history of infectious hepatitis does not necessarily bar organ donation. Surgeons recently have reported successful transplantation of kidneys from cadavers and from live donors who had tested positively for hepatitis B surface antigen.[27] There is no danger of contracting hepatitis from such donors if organ recipients are given hyperimmune globulin plus a booster dose of vaccine at the time of transplantation.

Contrary to a few opinions I've heard, not all potential recipients are averse to taking organs from condemned criminals. In 1988, I spoke with an eighteen-year-old man who had a transplanted liver, and to a thirty-four-year-old woman who had received a kidney from her living sister. Both of them had no reservations about accepting donations from death row and neither shuddered at the thought. If only a single patient among the thousands now awaiting donor organs wants to accept such a donation, then society and the medical profession are morally obligated to see that it is proffered.

Even though the medical community is loathe to act in that regard, it is unfair to blame individual doctors indiscriminately. After all, their politicized leaders control a powerful press that has succeeded in guiding most doctors into narrow channels of thought and behavior, especially in social and economic matters. Ambivalence among some of them is to be expected when inculcated authoritarian norms clash with their almost instinctive personal convictions. Many of the negative comments made in connection with my proposal are uttered by doctors afflicted in this way.

With that in mind, I performed another little test in 1984 on the American medical press, which has consistently rejected most of my articles and refused to abstract those published in a legitimate foreign journal. This time I tried the simpler "Letters-to-the-Editor" route. I summarized my proposal within the stipulated number of words and sent it to the editor of the highly respected *New England Journal of Medicine*. Predictably he rejected it in January 1985, citing as reasons the limited amount of space available for correspondence as well as his "judgment to present a representative selection of the material received."

Now, any sane reader of that journal's "Correspondence" section cannot help but question the sincerity of the editor's reply. Surely somewhere among the occasional witty poems, cute anecdotes, and mere personal palaver on strictly parochial issues—which consume a considerable chunk of that limited space—can be found a tiny niche for one short letter on a topic weighty enough to cut through the heart of many disciplines, particularly if that one letter *is* the entire representative selection.

I am not alone in voicing criticism. When in 1967 Dr. Maurice H. Pappworth, a member of the Royal College of Physicians, was preparing a book exposing numerous examples of flagrantly unethical medical practice and research, his colleagues urged him to refrain from such wide public exposure by publishing his findings in medical journals instead, thereby "keeping it in the family" so to speak. In the preface of his book Pappworth decried the fact that the "worst kind of experiments" are ignored because they tend to be published in journals having no correspondence columns. And, he continued, such columns as do exist generally are devoted only to discussions about "mundane, material matters of pay, status, and terms of service."[28]

Rejection of my letter manifested contravention of the *New England Journal of Medicine's* theoretical policy, proclaimed in 1986, as "a service to our readers to offer thoughtful commentary on social, economic, legal, and ethical issues facing the profession, (as) . . . an open forum responsive to responsible opinion on all sides of an issue."[29] There may be some measure of misrepresentation here, in view of the fact that Judge Amnon Carmi, the noted Israeli editor of *Medicine and Law*, considered my opinions to be responsible and thoughtful enough for publication in his indexed international journal.

It should be borne in mind that organ donation is but one facet of my proposal, albeit the most alluring and of immediate utility. Donation constitutes the most cogent reason for implementing the concept without delay and the most invincible obstacle for opponents. But the other facet, the basis of my original proposal in 1958, entails medical experimentation that, in the long run, is of infinitely greater value.

The choice of experimentation should always be available to any condemned convict—either as a routine option or, most importantly, as the *only* option for those who are too old to be organ donors. Their intact, live, anesthetized bodies would thereby offer invaluable opportunities for research in organ transplantation, for example, where animals are now sometimes being used. Or, that scenario would permit actual hands-on experience for surgeons in training or in pursuing new and difficult techniques.

These extraordinary circumstances call for an even better, more humane and well-controlled method of execution: routine general anesthesia, exactly as performed thousands of times every day in hospitals across the country, and induced at the instant set for the execution to begin. This is the *optimal* way to put a judicially condemned human to death, not only because it facilitates experimentation, but also because it permits the culling of all available vital organs in the best possible biological condition. Is it so barbaric or cruel to demand that society and the medical profession extend to condemned human beings the opportunity to die in a way extolled by surgeons as beneficent but now reserved solely for the animals they condemn to die in their research laboratories?

Evidently some of our most respected medical organizations, those with the most to gain from such a step and which ought to be the most strongly motivated to take it, think it is all that, and worse. Otherwise, why would my fervent pleas in 1982 for support from the American Association of Neurological Surgeons and from the International Anesthesiology Research Society go unanswered? Yet, innumerable cats, dogs, and monkeys continue to be nonchalantly sacrificed, as though no moral travesty were being committed.

Philosophical debility among doctors is even more pernicious and widespread than I had guessed. In his autobiography Nobel laureate Dr. Werner Forssmann prophesied that the increasing demand for transplantable organs will "pervert the concept of atonement" by resulting in the clamor for reinstatement and extension of the death penalty. He foresaw the depravity of prisons being turned into aseptic, hospital-like "organ banks" where executioners will be replaced by surgeons and anesthetists "degraded to the role of . . . Lucifer, Fallen Angel." [16]

Similar emotional "arguments" have been made by others. But they overlook the fact that the same objections were raised when the concept of gleaning organs from the clinically brain-dead was first introduced. A few panicky ethicists then raised the specter of wholesale unplugging of respirators in hospital intensive care units in order to speed up the availability of scarce organs. Just as that scare tactic was proved wrong and failed to kill a valuable concept, so, too, should latter-day alarmists like Dr. Forssmann be ignored when they predict that my proposal eventually will make death rows into the gigantic "organ farms" of their tortured imaginations.

In the same autobiography published in 1974, when organ transplantation was a fledgling temporarily grounded by insurmountable technical problems, Dr. Forssmann manifested dubitable foresight in weighing the envisioned ethical implications and psychological impact of heart transplantation, which he felt were "immensely ominous."[16] Time has proved his foresight flawed and his fear groundless: the public is now tremendously receptive to transplants, the practice is anything but ominous, and the ethical implications are less than wrenching. I have no doubt that Dr. Forssmann's attitude toward obtaining organs from death row will turn out to be equally unfounded and unjustifiably repressive.

It is sad irony that in his old age Dr. Forssmann seems to have petrified into the Dr. Sauerbruch of his youth.

10

Nothing New Under the Sun

The mid-morning coffee break at the University of Heidelberg seminar was a welcome respite from the coldly scientific description of charts, graphs, and photomicrographs. It was October 1983 and the first day of an international seminar on "Methods of Cerebral Blood Flow and Metabolism Measurement in Man." With a fresh donut and a cup of hot coffee in hand, I strolled aimlessly along the spacious hallway toward the lobby of the Pathologisches Institut and happened to stop by a door bearing a sign: "Prof. Dr. Wilhelm Doerr, Prof. Emer. of Pathology." Maybe the professor might be able to give me some sorely needed information, I thought, so I decided to extend my coffee break and inquire.

For several months I had been planning an article on the history of experimentation on condemned and executed humans, but my search of the literature in the United States—including the Library of Congress—had not been very productive. When writing up my original proposal back in 1958, I had felt uneasy about submitting a paper for publication without citing any relevant documented work other than second-hand references to the Alexandrians. Intuition told me that direct documentation could be buried in archives somewhere in the world, and I hoped that the professor might lead me to it.

This was not the first time that I faced such a problem. In 1960, at the Pontiac (Michigan) General Hospital, when the results of the first phase of our cadaver blood transfusion research were ready for publication, we had only the articles previously published by Russian investigators to cite as references. Only after our paper had been accepted for publication in 1961 did we learn of a similar study done by a surgeon, Dr. Leonard Charpier, in Chicago in 1935.[30] Unfortunately his experience was not documented in a medical journal at that time and therefore did not show up in a literature search. After a doctor in Central America read our report, he told us that cadaver blood transfusions had been performed there in a small regional hospital, and the results had been published in the institution's own provincial and obscure journal, which was not in the purview of indexed literature and therefore inaccessible. These revelations drove home to me the truth of the adage that there really is "nothing new under the sun."

In that frame of mind, I gave in to my propensity for unannounced intrusion and entered Professor Doerr's office. The reception was surprisingly cordial—a far cry from the old "Herr Professor" image. Luckily the professor, too, was interested in the topic of experimentation on condemned individuals and had a couple of references immediately in mind. He jotted them down, and in return for the favor asked only that I send him a copy of my paper if and when published. A quick glance at his note assured me that the cited German journals were available at many medical school and hospital libraries in the United States. And the titles of the articles suggested research that would expand the meager material I had already accumulated into an article of respectable length and content.

Once back in Michigan I browsed through the stacks of the

Shiffman Medical Library at Wayne State University in Detroit for the first article by a Dr. J. Henle in 1887, but it was not available. However, with the help of Library Director Faith Van Toll I found the second reference, which had been published in 1906 in the *Zeitschrift für experimentelle Pathologie und Therapie*: it was titled "Observations on the Isolated Surviving Human Heart." This was a very detailed report in which the authors described similar studies published more than a decade earlier, including those by Henle. At last I had enough material for what I believed would be a paper worthy of a journal of medical history.

I had been impressed by a copy of the *Medizinhistorisches Journal* from Germany, so I sent my manuscript to its editor, Prof. Dr. Gunter Mann, head of the Institute of Medical History at the University of Mainz. A couple of months later my paper was returned with Prof. Mann's cordial letter of rejection and an enclosed copy of his own latest publication.[12] The latter was a comprehensive monograph which more than reinforced what he said in the letter: that my presentation was far too superficial from an historical point of view to qualify for publication in his journal. Even though my effort included all that was then available to me, his exhaustive work dealing with an isolated historical example in and around Mainz, and supported with an extensive list of references, convinced me that he was right. I was grateful for this rich source of material to add to what I had on hand and thereby help fill a void in the medical literature in English.

Now I was faced with the question of where to submit my expanded paper entitled, "A Brief History of Experimentation on Condemned and Executed Humans." I realized that it still was not "academic" enough to please the fastidious editors of journals devoted exclusively to historical research. On the other hand, because I had no academic credentials and because the subject of my paper is anathema to medical authorities, I knew that it would never be accepted by editors of so-called prestigious journals.

Therefore, to spare myself time and aggravation, I decided—correctly—to submit it to the less prestigious but equally reputable *Journal of the National Medical Association*.[31] The article represented the most comprehensive history of the topic ever published in medical journals in the United States, if not the world, and should provide professionals and laymen alike more than enough information to satisfy their interests.

Historically the earliest association of medicine and condemned humans is obscure. We can only guess at it. Despite the lack of documented evidence, some scholars assume that the ancient Greeks of Homer's time, about 3,000 years ago, gained medical knowledge through the ritual sacrifice of human beings as "food" for their pagan gods. It is the high quality of medical references in Homer's works that led to the assumption.

But the assumption is tenuous because there was a universal dread of corpses and of other powerful religious and magical taboos among ancient peoples. So other historians, with equal validity, deny that dissection or experimental handling of candidates for ritual sacrifice was possible. Yet, these critics concede that knowledge of anatomy might have been gained through observation and treatment of wounds sustained in combat.

The case for experimentation on condemned criminals in Hellenistic Alexandria (ca. 300–200 B.C.) is more compelling, despite the fact that here, too, direct proof is lacking. In all likelihood that first golden age of science simultaneously nurtured the development of both postmortem dissection and vivisection. The pioneering Alexandrians probably were influenced by contact with neighboring Egypt, where the tradition of embalming provided excellent opportunities to explore the structure and relationships of internal body parts. But there is no evidence that the ancient Egyptians acquired any coherent or scientifically valid concept of anatomy from the practice.

We can trace Alexandria's enlightened atmosphere to the intense curiosity of the ruling kings, especially Ptolemy I Soter (367–283 B.C.) and his son Ptolemy II Philadelphus (308–246 B.C.). For the first time in recorded history they permitted and even encouraged public dissections. The Ptolemies themselves occasionally participated in the anatomic laboratories.

Because of this extremely lenient attitude, adherents of the dogmatic school of philosophy, which was dominant at the time, shifted their attention from static anatomy to the body's living processes. Here two giants are said to have performed medical experiments on living humans on a scale unmatched in history. They were Herophilus of Chalcedon (335–280 B.C.) and Erasistratus of Cos (c. 304–250 B.C.).

Herophilus, the older of the two, is conceded to be the father of anatomy. He believed in Hippocrates' humoral theory of health and disease. In addition to describing nerves, tendons, vessels, and many organs, Herophilus studied circulation of the blood and introduced many new drugs. His compatriot, Erasistratus, is known as the father of physiology. Rejecting the Hippocratic system, he extended the anatomic observations of Herophilus and delved into the function of blood vessels, capillaries, and heart valves.[32]

Historians assume that the Ptolemies forced condemned criminals to submit to experiments because these prisoners owed society a great debt and there was always a need for additional medical knowledge. Regrettably, this assumption is all we have, because the earliest evidence of the practice is indirect, from Roman historians writing 400 years later. These scholars accuse Herophilus and Erasistratus of having performed up to 600 vivisections, but much of the evidence on which the Roman historians based their accusations is now lost. This means that details about the subjects, whether or not anesthesia of some kind was used, and about the information obtained—all of which would support the historical claims—are missing.

Nevertheless, the historians' best guess is that live human experimentation was indeed practiced on a grand scale when the dogmatists predominated in Alexandria. If their guess is wrong, it means that the historians Celsus and Tertullian invented the fiction to spice up their treatises for their fellow Romans, but that is unlikely: both historians repudiated the practice of opening live bodies to observe nature at work. Tertullian went so far as to call the two Alexandrian scientists fanatical butchers. Celsus' criticism was milder; he thought it better to get the facts from cadavers or from examination of wounds. This was a method the physician and medical writer Galen (130?–200?)

later raised to an art called *vulneraria speculatio*, "the contemplation of wounds."

The dogmatists' philosophy created an ideal milieu for vivisection. Their preference for the study of function drove them to experiment on living persons, not out of sadistic curiosity, but rather in the serious pursuit of biologic truth. As far as they were concerned the potential suffering of a few social debtors could not outweigh the great benefit thereby bequeathed to future generations.

Furthermore, the dogmatists questioned the wisdom of applying the results of animal studies to man. At this time condemned criminals ranked with animals in the social order, and, in addition, all Alexandrian citizens were losing their status through gradual disenfranchisement. This trend inevitably led to contempt for the mortal body and exaltation of a soul that doomed criminals were supposed to have forfeited.

Some historians continue to doubt that Herophilus and Erasistratus actually took part in the scientific slaughter of 600 criminals. One good reason is that Galen, who often opposed the views of Erasistratus, never mentioned it. Celsus repudiated vivisection as being cruel and useless. He said that it defeats its own purpose because immediately after the body is opened, the color, texture, and other qualities of body parts differ from those in an untouched state. Consequently, all traces of human vivisection in Alexandria vanished along with the dogmatists.

Shortly thereafter, the scene shifted to ancient Pergamum in northwest Asia Minor, where the king, Attalus Philómetor, a contemporary of Cato (234–149 B.C.), was preoccupied with the nurture and study of poisonous plants. He tested various toxic plants and antidotes on condemned criminals. Unfortunately, no further details were included in the report.

With the rise of Rome all scientific human dissection disappeared from the Western world. Roman physicians could occasionally supplement their knowledge through treatment of wounded gladiators and through access to the mutilated bodies of criminals condemned to die under the attack of starved wild beasts as part of the infamous Coliseum games. But serious human experimentation remained dormant for over a thousand years. It surfaced again in the thirteenth century in a manner which few would have dared imagine, and in a land which fewer still had even heard of.

Greater Hyke (Cilician Armenia) was that land, where the first documented evidence was encountered with reference to the same practice that Celsus and Tertullian had attributed to the Alexandrians and had vehemently denounced.[33] According to the thirteenth-century Armenian philosopher-scientist, Hovhannes Yerzengatsi, and his teacher, Vartan Areveltsi, criminals condemned to death in medieval Armenia were vivisected for the purpose of not only studying the complexity of human anatomy, but also searching for better ways of treating and preventing disease. This was confirmed by another article based on a thirteenth-century account published by Vahram Rabbunu.[34] It describes studies on the heart, liver, intestines, and blood vessels, involving direct observations on condemned criminals. Rabbunu's competence and reputation added much weight to Yerzengatsi's report.

Still a third reference appeared in 1977,[35] again confirming Yerzengatsi's work and adding that it was, in part, reiteration of earlier documentation by Areveltsi, and even earlier by Areveltsi's teacher, Hovhannes Vanagan, who died in the year 1251. According to this account, the vivisection of condemned prisoners was a practice unique to Greater Hyke and aimed primarily at studying blood vessels and circulation, and their relationship to other body parts. The subjects apparently were weakened by starvation and given plenty of wine to drink before the experiments. There was no specific information about consent on the part of the subjects or how insensitive the wine made them.

This evidence, however, supports my guess that criminals in Ptolemaic Alexandria also were somehow benumbed before vivisection. It is difficult to imagine how any reasonably productive experiment could be carried out until the criminal was in alcoholic coma. Furthermore, it is known that Pedianus Dioscorides, a doctor in Nero's army in the first century A.D., used mandrake* to induce sleep before operations. He was familiar with local, general, and even rectal

---

*A poisonous plant.

anesthesia—and, in fact, is said to be the first to have used the word "anesthesia."[36]

Was vivisection unique to Greater Hyke? Probably not. At the same time the dissection of cadavers was being revived in pre-Renaissance Europe by daring anatomists who risked the wrath of a superstitious populace further outraged by widespread body snatching. Because of provincial isolation and poor means of communication, the audacious Armenians might not have known of another exception to the otherwise universal abhorrence of human vivisection. That exception was France, where the practice was described a little more than a century after the Armenian documentation.

King Louis XI (1461–1483) asserted that a condemned criminal should not be executed before contributing something to science. We don't know if the criminal was consulted, but by royal decree any reputable surgeon could experiment on a criminal facing imminent execution. Accordingly, the throne and the entire royal court often went to a nearby cemetery to observe the itinerant surgeon dissect a usually nude and fully conscious criminal tied to a slab beside a freshly dug grave. The surgeon treated witnesses to a running commentary on the functions of the parts being dissected. As a rule, the prisoner remained conscious long enough to see his own intestines dangled before him, and the lecture ended with his death. Historians say that significant scientific knowledge was gained from these excruciating executions and that Louis's medical patronage was widely acclaimed throughout Europe.[10]

One specific case was typical.[37] A thief, called the Archer of Meudon, who suffered from symptoms attributed to kidney stones, was condemned to die on the gallows of Montfaulcon near Paris in 1474. His crime was the sacrilege of stealing from the church. Many villagers, including high officials, also suffered from similar symptoms, and local surgeons decided to resume operations on the kidney, which had been abandoned in Europe but were still a part of Arabian medicine.

When the Archer's judicial appeal was rejected, King Louis XI placed him at the disposal of surgeons eager to test their skills. The incision accidentally opened the peritoneal cavity to expose loops of bowel, which the surgeons replaced. If a stone was actually seen or removed, there was no mention of it. The criminal survived the ordeal; and, not surprisingly, there were fewer complaints throughout the region of symptoms due to kidney stones.

An occasional unsubstantiated accusation of vivisection cropped up in the next century. Berengarius, having been falsely accused of vivisecting humans in Italy in 1521, vindicated himself by explaining that his *anatomia vivis* ("living anatomy") was knowledge gained through routine surgery (*anatomia fortuita*) and through *vulneraria speculatio*. What probably happened was that during either surgery or mere observation, the anguished cries of patients undoubtedly had been misinterpreted by horrified and superstitious laymen.[38]

About the same time (1564) the immortal anatomist, Andreas Vesalius, made a pilgrimage to Jerusalem. It was rumored to have been in penance for performing an accidental vivisection. According to a letter written shortly after Vesalius's death, while serving as court physician for Emperor Charles V of Spain, the great anatomist started to perform an autopsy on a young nobleman who had apparently died of a baffling disease. On opening the chest Vesalius was said to have been horrified to see the subject's heart still beating. The subject's parents wanted to charge Vesalius with impiety so that he would suffer the harshest punishment meted out by the Inquisition. But the emperor intervened to save him if he went to the Holy Land for atonement.[39] There is no factual basis for this story, which probably arose from Vesalius's prior well-known reputation for dissecting bodies of executed criminals.[40]

A vivisection controversy still surrounds one of Vesalius's most famous pupils, Fallopius, who was professor of anatomy at Pisa. In his book published in 1563, Fallopius tells how the Duke of Tuscany gave him custody of a condemned man to do with as he wished. The criminal was suffering from quartan fever,* and Fallopius wanted to test various therapeutic doses of opium. He started with three drams†

---

*A recurring fever at four-day intervals.

†One dram = one-eighth ounce.

when the prisoner was suffering a paroxysm* of fever. It had no effect. The criminal was willing to undergo another trial with the hope of winning a pardon from the duke. Fallopius gave the criminal another three-dram dose—but this time during a remission of symptoms—and the patient died.[41]

Two centuries later, Fallopius's experiment was harshly criticized as having been comparable to what were then called the atrocities of Alexandria. Critics in the eighteenth century deemed it incredible that a Christian physician could be so "barbaric" in so enlightened a time.[42] A different historical account dismisses the entire affair as extreme overreaction to Fallopius's well-known zeal for research. But the old professor's own words—which I have read—prove that he really did perform the experiments.

Meanwhile, during one or two centuries after the time of Fallopius, the public and medical profession in Europe gradually came to tolerate and, at times, even encourage scientific experimentation in connection with the death penalty. Some cases involved doctors of high standing in royal courts. One of them was William Cheselden, a prominent eighteenth-century English doctor appointed Surgeon Extraordinary to Queen Caroline. He was famous for performing lightning-fast operations for bladder stones in the era of surgery without anesthesia. He was also interested in research on the eye and the ear. Because the queen was hard of hearing, Cheselden suggested in 1743 that removal of part of the eardrum might cure her.

A criminal was to be executed around that time, and the court granted Cheselden's request to have the death sentence commuted if the criminal agreed to submit to the experimental surgery. Of course, the criminal consented. But the public, clamoring only for revenge, would have no part of it; and the court was forced to reverse itself. The decision deprived Cheselden of the only opportunity to test his idea.[43]

Almost a half-century later, again in England, Edward Jenner (1749–1823) revealed his formula for smallpox vaccine. But the pub-

---

*A convulsion or severe spasm.

lic was wary of the vaccine because some unscrupulous and ignorant doctors had caused localized outbreaks of the disease by using impure batches contaminated with the smallpox virus. So, then Princess Caroline ordered the vaccine tested on six condemned criminals to prove it safe for use on her own children.[28]

Across the channel, thoughts were turned toward making the death penalty more civilized. Humanitarian concern over the ends and means of prisons and capital punishment first emerged in Continental Europe. The movement was fueled by famous eighteenth-century intellectuals, such as Voltaire, Montesquieu, and Beccaria.

The penal reform that followed did not abolish the death penalty, which seemed to be as indispensable then as it is in our day; and in keeping with their egalitarian posture, Parisian legislators strove to make executions uniform and as infallible as possible for aristocrats and commoners alike. They and all French citizens knew that beheading sometimes resulted in needless suffering, especially when the victim was uncooperative, the sword or ax was wielded incompetently, or the blades were dulled by repeated use. They agreed that some sort of reliable mechanical device was needed. Its most ardent advocate was Dr. Joseph Ignace Guillotin,[44] who, at the age of fifty-one, had been elected in 1789 to serve along with seventeen other elected doctors as a deputy in the 1,200-member National Assembly.

Contrary to an almost universal misconception, Guillotin did not invent or participate in the development or construction of the device that, to his everlasting dismay, eventually bore his name. He was merely its most enthusiastic supporter as the best means of achieving swift and painless justice in a uniform way. The infamous beheading machine was designed by another doctor, the Secretary of the Academy of Surgery and Surgeon to the Crown, Dr. Antoine Louis, in whose honor it was originally called "louisette."

Dr. Louis based his design on the Halifax gibbet that had been used in England and Scotland since 1307 and refined in the sixteenth century as the "Maiden" (which was the actual precursor of the louisette). A German harpsichord maker built the first model under Dr. Louis's close supervision.[6]

The model passed its first test on live sheep without a hitch. However, after several successful trials on lean male and female corpses borrowed from a nearby hospital, the originally flat blade stuck part-way through the thick neck of a very husky man. The setback forced Dr. Louis to experiment with various blade designs, even one, it is said, suggested by King Louis XVI, who later fell victim to his own ingenuity. Dr. Louis tested many shapes, including those with concave and convex cutting edges, and finally settled on the king's design—a blade with a straight but diagonal cutting edge. The latter functioned without mishap when used for the first time on a live human on 25 April 1792, and for many thousands of beheadings during the infamous Reign of Terror that followed. Guillotin was horrified and disgusted.

Notwithstanding the horror of this method of decapitation, it cannot be doubted that Drs. Guillotin and Louis were acting in sincere accord with the traditional medical mandate to ease the suffering of those to be killed by judicial decree. Their example stands in stark contrast to today's medical leaders who oppose lethal injection and deny its humaneness to the condemned.

Wholesale beheadings and important discoveries in electricity coincided in the late eighteenth century and led to unique experiments dealing with human physiology. Luigi Galvani's (1737–1798) concept of "animal electricity" had raised naive hopes that science was on the verge of uncovering the ultimate essence of life itself. This prompted feverish research on a catalog of theories centering around the moment of death. After extensive probes on sacrificed animals, investigators now took advantage of society's waxing tolerance of such experiments and turned to the extraordinary opportunities offered by judicial executions.

Most of these experiments entailed mere visual observation instead of objective measurements. One of the earliest took place in Germany in 1791 before a group of doctors and medical students assembled to witness an execution.[12] Immediately after the criminal was decapitated, the investigator demonstrated that muscles in the torso's neck quiver when touched with a probe. Deeper contact caused muscular contractions strong enough to arch the back and to spread out the arms that had been folded over the chest. A light touch of the probe on the cut end of the spinal cord (in the part of the neck attached to the head) evoked similar twitches in facial muscles, especially around the lips. At times the eyelids blinked. Deeper probing here caused massive contraction of all facial and tongue muscles. The grotesque grimaces caused a few shuddering observers to turn away and leave. The startling consensus: consciousness probably persisted after decapitation.

The same conclusion was reached by another German investigator who used electrical stimulation to cause contractions in muscles in the severed heads of men and animals. The controversy over the possible persistence of consciousness deepened and led to similar experiments in other leading nations of Europe. At the Hôtel-Dieu in Paris the famous Dr. Marie François Bichat (1771–1802) was among the first to study the effects of electricity on guillotined criminals.

From Turin came a report of electrical stimulation performed in August 1802 by Italian doctors on the bodies of three beheaded criminals—again, before a large audience.[45] The first experiment began twenty minutes after execution. One pole of an electrical voltaic pile was connected with the torso's spinal cord, the other with the surface of the exposed heart. The latter contracted strongly and continued to contract even after the circuit was broken. (In a way, this experiment anticipated electrical cardioversion used today to restart the heart of certain patients.) Testing on the other two bodies only five minutes after beheading yielded even more vigorous contractions. When the aorta and other large arteries were filled with warm water and stimulated, they too contracted strongly. Heart reaction disappeared in about forty minutes, but the voluntary muscles continued to contract for a longer period.

In January 1803 authorities in England permitted a visiting Italian doctor to demonstrate his previous research on the body of a twenty-six-year-old man who had been hanged. The body remained outdoors in freezing temperature for an hour before being taken to a nearby laboratory equipped with an electrical pile of paired copper and zinc plates immersed in acid. When one electrode was put on an ear of the corpse and the other on a lip, the jaws quivered and one eye opened. Next, the electrodes were attached to both ears, and all muscles contracted, the slightly protruding tongue pulled back, and the entire head moved. The response to an ear-rectum circuit was so strong that the onlookers thought the body was coming back to life.

The same Italian investigator had done prior testing on severed heads in Bologna. There he had noted that electrical contact on the lips caused a small amount of saliva to flow from the mouth. When touched to the exposed surface of the brain, all facial muscles reacted. Direct contact of the electrodes to the optic and olfactory nerves gave no reaction. Instead of supplying answers to the question of persistence of consciousness in severed heads, this kind of experimentation merely polarized the controversy and broadened the scope of activity.

Those who insisted that consciousness did persist in a severed head—for even up to a quarter of an hour—were encouraged by results from an execution in Breslau, Germany, on the morning of 25 February 1803.[46] Immediately after the criminal was beheaded by sword, an electrical device produced strong muscular contractions in the head. Two assistants then held the head firmly while the researcher stared intently at the face. At the same time the cut end of the spinal cord was touched with a mechanical probe. The facial muscles contracted and the lips twisted. It looked like a grimace of pain. When the researcher swiftly thrust his finger toward the open eye of the detached head, its lids closed as though the brain were conscious of an immediate threat. The eyelids also closed when the head was faced toward the sun.

Next, the investigator shouted the victim's name into an ear. The eyelids opened, and the gaze slowly turned toward the source of the sound. The mouth made movements as though trying to open and speak. A local merchant who was timing the various phases of the experiment announced that one and a half minutes had elapsed at the end of the hearing test.

Galvanic stimulation was repeated, and muscular reaction was now weaker. However, deep mechanical probing of the spinal cord yielded facial contortions so violent as to cause many to shout, "He's alive!"

The eyelids slammed shut, and they were further compressed by muscular spasms that puffed the cheeks as though in pain. Teeth clamped down on fingers inserted into the mouth of the severed head, and even more forcefully with repeated probing of the spinal cord. Another independent experiment of this kind in the same years revealed traces of muscular activity for more than an hour after decapitation.

On the other hand, many of these observations were contradicted in experiments performed several months later, in Mainz, on seven of twenty criminals executed by guillotine on 21 November 1803.[12] The research team consisted of nine doctors and pharmacists and three medical students. Two of the latter, stationed directly beneath the scaffold, checked for evidence of consciousness immediately after decapitation. While one student picked up and held the head firmly with both hands for concentrated observation of the face, the other shouted in the ear, "Do you hear me?" Alternating tasks, they did this with seven heads. The eyelids, which never moved, initially varied from wide open to totally shut. The students noted no reaction in the eyes themselves. This team concluded that decapitation results in practically instantaneous and irreversible loss of consciousness.

A special two-room hut built on the site was equipped with electrical devices for experiments on the headless torsos. Five of the bodies were taken to the hut during an interval of from four to twenty-two minutes after beheading. In addition to doing routine electrical stimulation of muscles and nerves, the researchers injected a resinous fluid into the body cavities and applied charges to determine if there was any change in the ability of the blood and lymphatic vessels to absorb the fluid. No change was recorded.

Eye dissection after the electrical experiments revealed that cataracts had been liquefied. This raised hopes that electrical stimulation might be a new cataract treatment. But the finding could not be confirmed by others, and it became just another topic of dispute being aired in newspapers in connection with the relative merits of hanging and beheading.

As already discussed in chapter 4, the bitter controversy over the persistence of consciousness after execution by either of those two methods posed an insoluble dilemma. Even the king of Prussia acknowledged this in April 1803 in his letter to the chancellor. It was the king's opinion that experiments on beheaded men merely proved the existence of muscular contractility but not the persistence of consciousness. He said that only incontrovertible evidence would cause him to change the method of execution.

These studies on guillotined criminals may seem to have been unduly macabre, but in reality they were in line with the ethics of those times. The status of the condemned in the eighteenth and nineteenth centuries was about the same as that of capital offenders in ancient Alexandria. Regarded as little more than animals, condemned criminals still were deemed sufficiently more valuable than animals as instruments of research; and in that way they could make real restitution to society.

Authorities concluded that it made more sense to use the bodies of executed criminals for research than to comply with the medieval custom of merely leaving them to the ravages of exposure or of predatory beasts. Like the dogmatists who preceded them, eighteenth-century researchers insisted that human subjects were indispensable in certain fields of investigation (human consciousness, for example) if fundamental biological errors, such as the enduring ones fostered by Galen's animal studies, were to be avoided.

The experiments continued nevertheless, and led to the imposition of some restraints. In 1803 the Prussian king demanded that local authorities enforce strict rules for doctors applying for permission to experiment on beheaded criminals. He advised them to pay closer attention to the aims, the implications, and the repulsive nature of such research.[46]

Tighter control did not mean abolition, however. In fact, a few years later it was permissible to experiment on condemned men even before execution—usually with their consent. Many convicts were eager to submit in the hope of getting lighter sentences or outright pardons. But the granting of such favors was not universally endorsed. The philosopher Immanuel Kant and the physiologist Claude Bernard were among those who did not favor pardoning the survivors of research.

For Kant, "justice would cease to be justice, if it were bartered away for any consideration whatsoever."[47] And although Bernard opposed direct experimentation on condemned criminals, he approved of the removal and use of organs and tissues after decapitation.[48]

Despite Bernard's opposition, a few French doctors continued to do research on prisoners prior to execution. In 1834 an anonymous investigator injected himself with material taken from a plague victim in order to describe and understand details of the disease. To extend and broaden the scope of his study, he requested permission to use live condemned men; and five criminals volunteered. Specific information about the experiment is lacking. Four criminals survived to be executed. One died before execution, but it is not certain that the experiment was the cause.[49]

Again in France, a condemned woman was the subject of tapeworm research without her consent or knowledge.[50] Cysticerci (tapeworm larvae) were obtained from a pig and separated into groups of twelve to eighteen larvae. Mixed with sausage and soup, the larvae were fed to her in five meals during a seventy-two hour period before her execution. An autopsy was performed two days after her death. There were four young tapeworms in the duodenum* but the head of only one of them had a complete set of hooklets. Six more worms outside of the duodenum had no hooklets.

Critics doubted that the worms seen at autopsy came from the ingested larvae. They pointed out that the first group of larvae was fed to her sixty-four hours after having been taken from the pig, and that, in their opinion, was too long a time outside of a host's body for the larvae to survive.

Elsewhere in Europe executions were being exploited for the study of cardiac physiology. According to a German report in 1852,[51] for fifteen minutes the heart of a guillotined criminal showed spontaneous and rhythmic contraction in the right atrium and similar but weaker activity in the right ventricle. The left side was motionless. Repeated electrical stimulation of the heart stopped the contractions intermit-

---

*Small bowel just beyond the stomach.

tently, but action always returned. Amazingly it got stronger thirty-five minutes after decapitation, while an autopsy was going on. Observers concluded that it was due to the reflux of blood into the heart from abdominal organs being manipulated during the autopsy.

French investigators made similar observations a few years later.[51] The heart of a thirty-eight-year-old man guillotined in 1887 showed ventricular contractions lasting for twenty-five minutes, and for sixty-five minutes in the atria. On the other hand, after another decapitation in Paris in 1892, cardiac activity was totally absent during forty-five minutes of observation. Mechanical and electrical stimulation did nothing.

Then, for the first time on a human heart, the researchers tried resuscitative maneuvers perfected eleven years earlier on animal hearts. These involved infusing nutritive fluids into the coronary circulation. It was discovered that weak heart contractions could be evoked one hour after beheading by inserting a small tube into the aortic arch and introducing defibrinated arterial blood* from a dog into the coronary vessels of the human heart. The resultant contractions, limited to the right side, measured 148 per minute in the atrium and 44 per minute in the ventricle; and they were strong enough to propel blood into the pulmonary circulation. The contractions tapered off twenty-three minutes later into the irregular tremors of fibrillation, but another infusion, this time of fresh dog's blood, jump-started the heart back into a regular beat.

Nineteenth-century researchers in the United States sometimes used black slaves.[52] In some respects the experiments were similar to the concentration camp atrocities of our time. The potential for crippling injury or death was entirely irrelevant. Fortunately, most procedures involved little danger or cruelty, and outright malice on the part of experimenters was rare. Some of the latter used these opportunities merely to gain fame, but most were sincerely interested in testing new treatments, in gaining more knowledge and competence, and in boosting the quality of care.

---

*Blood from which the fibrin (thin filamentous material that forms the mesh-work of a clot) is removed.

A few of the experiments were dramatic. In one appalling instance researchers kept a male slave in an open pit oven to test a new method for treating heat stroke. In contrast, another very useful experiment was carried out on a slave woman in Alabama to develop a better technique for repairing vesicovaginal fistulas.*

As the twentieth century opened, doctors again turned to guillotine victims in their efforts to answer two important and enduring questions. First, how can one be sure that death has really occurred and thereby avoid dreaded premature burial? Second, does consciousness ever persist in a severed head?

Shortly after Hermann Helmholtz invented the ophthalmoscope in 1851, a French doctor tried to answer the first question by examining the retinas of freshly guillotined criminals.[53] The same manuever was repeated by others in France as well as in various countries over the next century; and in 1956 it was the basis of my first attempt at research.[54] There was no doubt that certain vascular and color changes in the retina constitute the fastest, most reliable, and most inexpensive way to determine if the heart has stopped beating and, by inference, death—and perhaps the point at which death becomes absolutely irreversible.

Efforts to settle the consciousness-in-the-severed-head question took some bizarre directions. On 28 August 1906 French surgeon Dr. Ronald Marcoux was permitted to experiment on a condemned murderer named Margret.[11] According to the surgeon's written account, he was an ideal subject whose cool composure demonstrated a sincere willingness to have his body help science immediately after decapitation.

Margret's severed head landed flat on the cut neck in the basket. This helped prevent excessive hemorrhage and gave the doctor more time to make observations. The face immediately showed the pallor and the half closed eyelids characteristic of death. Intermittent muscular twitches lasted only for several seconds. Marcoux then leaned

---

*Artificial openings between the vagina and bladder caused by inflammation and tissue breakdown.

into the basket and called out the criminal's name. He was astounded to see the eyelids open immediately—as though awakening from a dreamlike state—and the eyeballs turn to gaze directly at him for ten to fifteen seconds. Instead of having a cadaverous and glassy stare, it seemed as though there was an attempt at actual visual communication. The eyelids then calmly closed.

But they opened again when his name was repeated closer to his ear. This time the eyeballs tracked Marcoux as he moved around to the side of the basket, and appeared to end by focusing a steady gaze up at the bloody blade. The lids then closed permanently. This amazing experiment added more fuel to the raging controversy over the humaneness of beheading. It led critics to declare the guillotine to be the agent of "a callous vivisection followed by premature burial."

Another intriguing case was reported in a French newspaper in 1907. When a criminal named Menesclou was guillotined, a Dr. Amirault immediately pumped blood from a live dog into the criminal's severed head. That caused the pallor of death to disappear. For a few seconds the criminal's lips began to move as though trying to open the mouth, and the facial expression was described as one of "shocked amazement." The doctor continued the extrinsic blood supply circulating for two hours. The results prompted him to conclude that "a heart has reactivated the living brain, and speech is a distinct possibility."[11]

Amirault, too, denounced the guillotine as a barbaric form of execution because, he said, "this head, separated from the body, listens to the voices of the crowd. The decapitated man senses himself dying as he looks up at the guillotine blade in full recognition of what has happened."

Meanwhile, other doctors concentrated on the physiology of the heart. A well-controlled and detailed experiment was carried out on the heart isolated from, but still in place and connected to, the body of a French woman guillotined in 1905.[51] It confirmed observations made a half century earlier: that weak but persistent contractions on the right side of the heart were strengthened as well as induced in the previously motionless left side by perfusing the organ with warm

Ringer's solution* thirteen minutes after decapitation. Contractions grew in strength when warm, defibrinated human blood was substituted for the Ringer's solution. This human experiment confirmed the results of many prior animal studies.

American doctors became involved in research on condemned men early in the twentieth century. Among the first projects was one dealing with the development of a plague vaccine. In 1905 Dr. R. P. Strong, then stationed in the Philippines and later to become a famous professor of tropical medicine at Harvard University, persuaded the governor to place forty-two condemned men at his disposal.[55] He injected them under the skin with increasingly concentrated doses of cultured and weakened plague organisms previously tested on guinea pigs and monkeys. Strong read a report of his findings at a meeting of the Manila Medical Society on 6 November 1905. The matter of prisoner consent was not mentioned, nor was it discussed in his article published a year later.

Another American, Dr. B. C. Crowell, collaborated with Strong on a second project dealing with beriberi† in 1912.[56] This time twenty-nine condemned Filipino criminals consented to take part after being promised unlimited quantities of cigars and cigarettes. The convicts were divided into four groups and fed varied diets for up to 115 days. An occasional death resulted from beriberi and heart failure, confirmed by gross and microscopic autopsy findings. The experiment demonstrated conclusively that polished rice lacks an essential nutritive element.

These American research projects in the Philippines were cited by German doctors in their own defense at the Nuremberg War Crimes Trials in 1947.[57] They pointed out that Strong's fame resulted, in part at least, from experiments involving condemned men.

In Ceylon (now Sri Lanka) in November 1923 six condemned criminals became ill while taking part in experiments requiring the ingestion of carbon tetrachloride, followed by purges of epsom salts.[58]

---

*A solution of sodium, potassium, and calcium chlorides, isotonic (pH 5–7.5).
†A disease caused by deficiency of vitamin B.

This project, details of which are not available, was denounced in the English press.

A rare and comparatively innocuous episode of human experimentation involved a forty-two-year-old murderer condemned to death in Utah in 1938.[59] At that time the state offered a choice between firing squad and hanging. The convict chose the former, saying, "I lived by the gun; I'll die by the gun." Prior to the execution, Dr. Stephen Besley, the prison's medical officer, asked the convict if he would permit an electrocardiograph (ECG) tracing to be made during the execution. The convict readily agreed and replied, "Nuts! I gotta kick the bucket anyway, don't I?" His coarse attitude belied hidden altruism because, for the first time in his life, he wanted to do something good for society. Therefore, he donated his eyes to an ophthalmologist in San Francisco and his body to the University of Utah.

The ECG wires were attached to the murderer's wrists and ankles as he sat in front of a wall, in a chair firmly anchored to the ground. A short distance away, four bullets and one blank cartridge were loaded into the firing chambers of five rifles aimed in his direction through small holes in a makeshift wall of black muslin sheets. Besley placed a small target over the the convict's heart, which now was racing at three times the normal rate. As the four bullets tore through his heart, it went into a spasm lasting four seconds. That was followed by a fifteen-second interval of uniform electrical activity during which a second spasm occurred, then complete electrical "silence."

The most recent, extensive, and well-known experiments on condemned humans were done by Nazi doctors during World War II. But the world has completely ignored the medical crimes committed by Turkish doctors during World War I. There are many similarities between these two horrendous examples of medical atrocities, historically separated by a mere generation in our own century.

First, the perpetrators themselves manifested identical behavior. For those doctors, loyalty to the party in power and to its political philosophy came before conventional medical ethics. According to evidence presented by V. N. Dadrian, professor of history at the State University of New York at Geneseo,[60] Drs. Behaeddin Shakir, Nazim, and Hamdi Suad were as ruthlessly efficient in pursuing the Ittihad Party's "final solution" of the Armenian Question in the Sultan's Turkey of 1915–1918 as were Drs. Josef Mengele, Sigmund Rascher, and Karl Gebhardt in pursuing the Nazi Party's "final Solution" of the Jewish Question in Hitler's Germany of 1939–1945.[60,61]

Second, both regimes resorted to mass murder by means of gassing in special "disinfection centers." The Ottoman doctors introduced the gas chambers that were later perfected in the Nazi concentration camps.

Third, in many instances the sadistic doctors performed the same kinds of experiments on helpless, nonconsenting, innocent victims, without anesthesia or any other measures to lessen pain or distress. For example, Turkish and Nazi health authorities dreaded the outbreak of typhus epidemics among their troops. In searching for a serum antidote, they experimented on their respective Armenian and Jewish subjects as part of a campaign of deliberate genocide. As a result of the typhus experiments alone, many hundreds of young Armenians died in the city of Erzincan in 1916; and many hundreds of Jews perished in Buchenwald during the last four years of World War II.

The Nazi medical atrocities seem a greater travesty because of the traditionally superior quality and sophistication of German medicine. Their experiments centered on three basic aims: (1) primarily military, such as protecting personnel against cold temperatures and freezing at high altitudes, during parachute jumps, and when immersed in water; (2) military as well as general medical, such as research on infectious diseases, fractures, and limb transplantation; and (3) personal satisfaction of certain SS officers who pressed for the refinement of means for killing masses of people, for mass sterilization, and for a copious supply of material for their bizarre biological collections of skin and skulls.[62]

There was one big difference between the otherwise almost identical Turkish and Nazi medical war crimes. Whereas not a single Turkish doctor was prosecuted or even arrested by the Allied powers after 1918, the Nuremberg Tribunal arrested and tried twenty-three German medical defendants and sentenced seven of them to die by hanging.

Among them was Hitler's personal surgeon, Karl Brandt, who requested to be allowed to submit to experimentation during execution instead of merely being hanged. The tribunal rejected his extraordinary (and very sensible) suggestion.[63]

These medical crimes apparently were such a horrendous discovery for the civilized world that, regrettably, they seem to have blunted reason and common sense with regard to the rational assessment of the use of condemned human subjects for research. In and of *itself* human experimentation can never be criminal or corrupt. Only those who perform it can be. Through blind passion society often mistakenly attributes the corrupt character of the doer to what was or is being done.

In short, medical experimentation on consenting humans was, is, and most likely always will be the laudable and correct thing to do. The "why" of it is beyond doubt. Only the circumstances under which it is done—the who, when, and how—can be wrong or "criminal." And that is strictly a matter of mores and prevailing ethics, and of the soundness, relevance, and enforceability of the rules of conduct they foster.

11

Stone-Age Ethics
for Space-Age Medicine

A legitimate, comprehensive, and universally valid code of medical ethics no longer exists. In fact, it never did.

What has traditionally passed for "ethics" among doctors is a vague body of unwritten rules of obscure origin that loosely prescribes professional etiquette among themselves and for their relationship with patients. This seemed to be enough in the days of rudimentary medicine, when the doctors' carefully nurtured aura of godliness reinforced the psychological impact of their herbal concoctions for superstitious patients.

But today's modern patients expect much more. Now stripped of self-assumed sanctimony, many doctors are almost panicking because the old rules don't work any more. The once haughty healers now look to the law, to clerics, to a growing army of latter-day ethicists, to hastily contrived ethics committees, and even to the public for guidance on when, how, and why to use the awesome power modern science and technology have placed at their disposal.

Ask any doctor why he or she does or does not do certain things in certain ways and chances are you'll hear the words "Hippocratic Oath." Then ask what that oath is, and be prepared for a few confident replies amid a welter of stammering and poorly disguised guessing. Next, ask the confident ones where the oath came from, and observe how, with diminishing confidence, they will tell you that it was formulated by Hippocrates in ancient Greece; fewer still may add that he lived in Cos in the fifth century B.C.

For the majority of doctors, especially those over the age of fifty, and for me until very recently, the oath was something occasionally mentioned in medical school but rarely studied in detail. Even casual comments about it never seemed to go beyond a few selective clichés. I never took the oath, and as far as I know it was never officially administered to my graduating class in 1952 at the University of Michigan. Indeed, it is now uncommon for any American medical faculty to insist that the oath be taken by graduating doctors. That alone renders suspect the hallowed oath's importance or relevance to modern medical practice.

My knowledge of the Hippocratic Oath stems almost exclusively from the exhaustive treatise written by the preeminent medical historian Ludwig Edelstein.[64] It was in another of his detailed articles that I was introduced in 1958 to the Alexandrian practice that undergirds my proposal. He and other historians doubt that Hippocrates really authored the oath. They believe that it is a summary distilled in the fifth century B.C. from parts of Hippocrates' writings (the so-called *Corpus Hippocraticum*) plus ideas espoused by minor pagan sects such as Pythagoreanism and Orphism.[31]

Pythagoreanism was a popular, puritanical, and very secret religion. Its dogma was stern and unbending. Pythagoreans were the only ones who unconditionally denounced the then widely prevailing practices of abortion, infanticide, euthanasia, and suicide. Many Pythagorean principles were adopted and eventually sanctified by the Judeo-Christian tradition now dominating the Western world. But there is a sharp difference between the fundamental attitudes of the old Pythagoreans and of the Christians who followed them. And failure to appreciate that difference is, to a large extent, responsible for misinterpretation of the oath and for much unnecessary controversy extending to our time.

As far as the Pythagoreans were concerned, nothing of a moral nature was involved. Therefore, they abstained from judging nonbelievers who continued to practice what for Pythagoreans was strictly taboo. (Contrast this attitude with that of fanatically judgmental tendencies of modern Christians.)

The remarkable tolerance of otherwise very fastidious Pythagoreans apparently reflected a consensus missing in our society. They generally conceded that society could not function properly if everybody were forced to behave in unswerving obedience to Pythagorean principles. But when Christians inherited the Pythagorean legacy, they forgot the consensus and transformed their tenets into inflexible dogma, from which brutally punitive secular and ecclesiastical laws were derived and applied indiscriminately to everyone, regardless of personal creed or aspirations. Much of this universally constrictive code of conduct persists today and seems to be at the root of many of our complex bioethical dilemmas.

The medical profession makes matters worse by reinforcing these constrictions through homage to high-sounding platitudes. As far as my proposal is concerned, most doctors in control of medical organizations and academic centers would say that it's unethical and wrong, because doctors should treat and heal, not kill. It's wrong, because doctors should not cause harm (*primum non nocere*), but should always act only for the benefit of the patient after assessing the risk/benefit ratio. And if pressed to cite the authority for all this, the doctors invariably invoke the Hippocratic Oath.

Let's see exactly what the oath has to say. Near the middle of the 240-word oath is this statement: "I will apply dietetic measures for the benefit of the sick according to my ability and judgment; I will keep them from harm and injustice." (In talking about or dealing with patients, doctors always consider doing no harm, but I have never heard a doctor talk about injustice in relation to his patients.) Of course, more than dietetic measures is inferred from the oath's stipulation; otherwise it would have little meaning today, when medical practice is understood to entail almost everything but dietetics.

After acknowledging the fact that an execution is a state mandated ending of human life, how could any highly educated doctor see any harm done to someone being executed by means of irreversible general anesthesia? An experiment performed or organs taken can cause the subject no distress. The only conceivable harm might be that inflicted during the induction of anesthesia. But the experience of thousands of patients undergoing surgery every day in our hospitals would attest to how ridiculous that contention is. Alas, there is one circumstance in which my proposal would indeed inflict "harm," and that is in the pride of bigoted critics suffering the "pain" of offended dogma.

The risk/benefit ratio criticism is just as absurd. How can there be any risk for a criminal who, by law, must be destroyed? Benefit is another matter. If we permitted the condemned to die as I propose, we make it possible to extract some advantage from wasteful personal extinction. We confer upon the criminal the autonomy of decision relative to his or her own death as well as to the involuntary deaths of the victims of crime. We also proffer the equally precious benefit of a last chance to express any residual sense of altruism. By endorsing and implementing the proposal, doctors can transform the meaningless risk/benefit ratio of conventional judicial executions into a ratio of incalculable positivity. In the process doctors can satisfy to the letter the full injunction of their hallowed oath: they can keep the "patients" (the condemned) from harm *and* injustice.

The fear of being seen as killers intimidates doctors. Some mistakenly try to equate with murder the act of executing a peacetime death sentence. But how can that be? The law defines murder as "criminal homicide . . . committed with malice aforethought, either express or implied, and committed recklessly under circumstances manifesting extreme indifference to the value of human life."[65] It is obvious that this cannot apply to a doctor who has been permitted to experiment on, or take organs from, a willing criminal being executed. In fact, the doctor's act would manifest the highest regard for the value of human life in the most emphatic sense.

Yet, even when convinced that it's not murder, most doctors still object. What they fail to appreciate is that neither killing nor homicide per se entails or implies criminal or unethical conduct. That would depend on the circumstances involved. For example, killing by a soldier in the performance of wartime duty is both legal and moral and is sometimes lauded as heroic. The gory killing of religious heretics in past centuries was legal, and regarded as so moral as to be an almost divine duty. Similarly, in the case of judicial executions the "killer" is that abstraction called the law; the human executioner is merely the agent of implementation.

A simple analogy makes the point clearer. Any criminal is imprisoned by the law, not by the guard or turnkey. They implement the law by facilitating and guaranteeing the curtailment of freedom stipulated by the law. In like manner, the law does the killing, not the executioner. Saint Augustine made that plain fifteen centuries ago when he wrote that "there is no breach of this commandment which says 'Thou shalt not kill', in the case of those who . . . representing in their person the power of the state, have put criminals to death."[66]

No doubt many doctors would still refuse to do it. However, this is not a question of what one *would* do, but what one *should* or *ought* to do. Doctors seem to be confusing ethics with psychology.[67]

The medical profession's current ambivalence, contradiction, and equivocation are sure signs that a coherent and reliable guide to proper conduct by doctors does not exist. Just look at medicine's ridiculously fluctuating ethical position with regard to abortion. It is clear that the profession has taken the philosophically prudent course of letting public opinion and legal statutes determine whether it is ethical for doctors to perform abortions. Before the 1973 U.S. Supreme Court decision, abortion was illegal and therefore unethical. That decision suddenly made it legal and, of course, ethical; and doctors began doing abortions on a grand scale.

Now, will a reversal of the Court's decision make abortion un-

ethical again? Can genuine ethics be so chimerical, so fickle, so aimlessly—almost recklessly—changeable, like the mentality of some scatter-
brained child?

The answer is yes—for those doctors who really don't care or
who conveniently overlook, or are ignorant of, this short, nagging
sentence in the oath they are otherwise so fond of citing: "I will not
give to a woman an abortive remedy." There's nothing doubtful or
ambiguous about that genuinely Pythagorean decree. Therefore, every
doctor who now performs abortions, anywhere in the world, is guilty of unethical conduct according to the oath, which says nothing
about the sanction of secular law.

The violation is compounded by the fact that fetuses are killed
without the benefit of direct anesthesia. This poses a dilemma for
those who accept the claim of some obstetricians that fetuses as young
as three months feel and react to pain. If that is true, then an abortionist could be guilty of not only infringing the Hippocratic injunction against killing a fetus, but also the one that exhorts him or her
to do no harm.

I take no sides in the abortion controversy, just as I remain neutral on capital punishment. I bring it up only to expose the slipshod,
knee-jerk approach of the medical profession to matters of ethics.

Like their abortionist colleagues, those surgeons who procure organs from clinically brain-dead patients commit similar ethical trav-
esties—probably without even being aware of it or caring much about
it. In spite of a continual debate over what constitutes infallible criteria for determining brain death, surgeons as a rule accept as their
guide the absence of electrical activity in the brain and brain stem.
At that point they feel justified in removing organs for transplantation.

It is at this stage that they begin "bending" the ethical rules by
striving to keep the subject's still living body in the best possible
condition. They do so not primarily for the sake of their brain-dead
patient, but to help satisfy their own pressing need for transplantable
organs, which are in critically short supply. Then these surgeons bend
the rules further when they remove organs from the donors' un-
anesthetized bodies. They assume that the brain's complete electrical

"silence" signifies total loss of all function. But tiny islands of sensory cortex could still be viable enough to sense some degree of pain when organs are removed. In that case the subjects' awareness of pain would be impossible to detect if the complete loss of the brain's motor function rendered the agonized subjects incapable of movement.

This critical but easily ignored point was emphasized by two British doctors who accuse some surgeons of grievously infringing medical ethics by neglecting to let dying potential organ donors know "that they may not be dead in their understanding at the time of organ removal."[68]

Doctors have ventured beyond simple organ procurement from comatose, brain-dead patients to the extreme of using them for risky research. It is not widely known that in 1983 an early model of a totally artificial heart was tried on five brain-dead patients in Philadelphia.[69] Three of the five were also kidney donors, and informed consent had been obtained from the patients' relatives for the donations as well as for the experimentation. The doctors wrote that "because of the unique *no risk* (italics added) situation of the subjects, the function of the artificial heart could be tested in a manner not advisable in patients, but necessary for clinical preparation. The subjects were placed on total cardiopulmonary bypass, but there was no mention of general anesthesia. The experiments lasted up to seventy-two hours, then the researchers quit to allow for funeral arrangements.

In April 1986 another experiment was reported in France on a young man who had been brain-dead for three years. It involved the rapid transfusion of blood into the man's pelvic bones. The experiment was condemned by a French bioethicist, but the head of a commission on anesthesia said he saw nothing wrong "if there is proof of brain death."[70]

The growing shortage of donor organs is miring surgeons more deeply in ethical ambivalence. Their cautious and sporadic use of tissues and organs from aborted fetuses and from live anencephalic infants* heralds an era of wholesale exploitation of these sources. This

---

*Deformed newborns having no brain.

has generated more controversies that, in the end, will probably serve very little purpose other than to guarantee the sinecures of many overpaid ethicists.

It should be obvious from the cited examples that contrary to their self-righteous objections, doctors do indeed kill—they kill condemned fetuses, infants born without brains, and living patients with dead brains.

Consider this paradox: doctors themselves arbitrarily decide when to take hearts, lungs, and livers, from comatose, brain-dead, but otherwise living subjects. They therefore kill innocent and gravely ill humans who are comatose *persons*; who owe no debt to society as, for instance, a condemned criminal does; and who are powerless to give direct consent. On the other hand, these same doctors refuse to act on behalf of a much higher authority than their own volition (the laws of society which condemn criminals and which might allow them to donate organs or submit to experiments)—an act which would be performed in a manner that is anything but arbitrary, and at a time carefully set by that higher authority. Furthermore, the condemned owe society an enormous debt and are perfectly healthy, conscious, and capable of giving reasoned and fully informed consent.

The ethical travesty doesn't stop here. Surgeons desperately searching for additional sources of organs have turned to animals. In the early 1960s a New York surgical team tried several times unsuccessfully to transplant chimpanzee kidneys into humans. In 1964 an adult patient at the University of Mississippi was given a chimpanzee's heart. And the use of a baboon's heart for Baby Fae in California was widely publicized in 1984.

Primate donors are expensive and relatively scarce, so surgeons are resorting to pigs as donors. Porcine tissues are remarkably similar to ours biologically and would seem to be ideal for heterologous (different species) transplantation of foreign organs (xenografts). Extensive research in this field is underway in Alabama, Minnesota, and New York where surgeons plan to implant pigs' hearts into humans in the very near future.[71]

Here we have another outrageous ethical infraction. Surgeons disregard the question of possible animal autonomy and wantonly sacrifice innocent and obviously disinterested "lower" creatures by killing them to obtain xenografts. At the same time, surgeons insist that it is "unethical" to take advantage of the clearly determinable autonomy of the condemned, who are both legally guilty and deeply indebted, can give informed consent, and want and need to offer far more desirable species-specific homografts that will otherwise be wasted.

How sad it is that misguided surgeons deem the greedy snatching of life from a sanitized sty full of condemned pigs to be more respectable and "moral" than accepting it graciously from a gloomy death row full of condemned humans.

An honest answer to a simple question will reveal the integrity of one's ethical outlook: if you needed a heart transplant, would you rather have the heart of a reluctant pig or that of a willing young condemned human being?

The example of the surgeons in Philadelphia demonstrates how muddled medical thinking has become in matters of ethics. Researchers are on ethical quicksand when they ignore inmates on death row and instead use sick patients for transplantation research. They act as though the condemned do not exist and are not being purposely destroyed— as though they would not serve as better subjects for experimentation than the innocent, debilitated patients who are forced to serve as "guinea pigs" when new procedures, drugs, and techniques are tried for the first time on humans.

A fine dissection of the Hippocratic Oath[64] will show why most of these infractions of ethics (and of common sense, too) are so prevalent. The few doctors who actually take the oath do so by swearing to a few of the pagan gods and goddesses of ancient Greece, thereby binding themselves to mythological deities about whom they know little and care nothing. Technically committed by oath, a doctor then has no business invoking any other principle or creed. Judeo-Christian ideas then become not only irrelevant but anathema.

Next, the oath directs the doctor to revere his teachers as his parents; to share his money with them; to regard their children as his; and to very secretly instruct his own and his teachers' sons, but only if they take the oath, and only them and nobody else. Most of this is patently silly today, and some of it downright immoral, if not illegal —such as the stipulated secrecy which would bar instructing the public on matters of personal and even public health.

The next clauses dealing with harm, injustice, and abortion have already been discussed. (Included here is a prohibition against giving patients deadly drugs, which is discussed in chapter 13.)

Taken literally, all doctors who do surgery violate the oath's ban on using the knife, "even on sufferers from stone," and therefore are unethical. Actually this injunction was meant for doctors who deal only with medicaments. In ancient times they were considered to be the only real doctors, because cutting was considered to be too crass an activity for their exalted station in life. That was left to the lower class barbers (so-called barber-surgeons). This distinction survives to our time in England, but in name only. Surgeons there take pride in being called "mister" instead of "doctor."

The oath stipulates dedication to benefiting the sick and to staying "free of all intentional injustice, of all mischief, of all sexual relations with both female and male persons." The first part is above criticism, but there are doctors who certainly do infringe the rest with all kinds of mischief —becoming alcoholics and drug addicts, doing unnecessary surgery or other treatments, performing risky research without consent, and having illicit sexual relations—even with patients and sometimes without their consent or ability to resist.

Toward its conclusion the oath binds doctors to keep their dealings with patients in strict confidence, which they continue to do scrupulously.

Finally, it has a stern warning for those who would breach the oath, and threatens them with dishonor and infamy "among all men for all time to come."

Most, if not all, doctors today couldn't care less about pagan gods to whom they are supposed to have sworn allegiance. Neither do they consider the sons of their teachers and other doctors to be theirs, and they wouldn't dream of sharing their money with their teachers. Some delight in reaping huge incomes from abortions and unnecessary surgery, in doing ethically questionable experiments as both peacetime and wartime atrocities, in being doped or drugged while treating patients, and in fornicating with them as a form of "therapy."

Of the roughly ten points comprising the Hippocratic Oath, at least seven were, and continue to be, violated on a significant scale. But worst of all, doctors cannot (or choose not to) enforce ethical behavior on their own. Only recently has the profession tried to begin a "house cleaning," but quite feebly and simply because it feels intimidated into doing so by public and governmental indignation.

Licenses to practice medicine are revoked in only a tiny percentage of cases of serious violation of laws, and rarely if ever for the violation of ethics alone. Delinquent doctors usually are put on probation or given some other mild "slap on the wrist" and allowed to go on practicing. None of these measures embodies the threat of the oath to shackle the wrongdoers with "eternal infamy and dishonor." But that is an empty threat, and it always has been, because human beings rarely fear a spiritual threat. Even Hippocrates knew that when in *The Law* he lamented that "there is no punishment connected with the practice of medicine (and with it alone) except disgrace; and that does not hurt those who are familiar with it."[72]

Many doctors admit that the oath is hopelessly outdated. In recent years several new codes have been concocted, such as the Declaration of Geneva in 1948 (amended at Sydney, Australia, in 1968); the Declaration of Helsinki in 1964 (amended in Tokyo in 1975); and in 1978 the U.S. Department of Health, Education, and Welfare Regulations on the Protection of Human Subjects.[73]

All of the new codes do little else than perpetuate clichés. None of them even addresses the issue of experimentation on doomed humans. That is especially deplorable in the case of the so-called Nuremberg Code, which was formulated to prevent future atrocities in that regard. It is incredible that the Nuremberg Tribunal in 1947 could be satisfied with a document that doesn't even mention what it was convened for in the first place!

It is not difficult to pinpoint the biggest reason for continuing unethical medical conduct and the often terrible tragedies it fosters. We can trace the causal thread way back to the dawn of the human race, when a very crude type of medical practice was the sole responsibility of those in control of the religious life of tribal communities. Progressing from them through the medical priests in Egyptian, Mayan, and Incan civilizations, and the powerful medieval European theocracies, to the persisting strong vestiges today, it is clear that the medical profession has been unable or unwilling to rid itself of the now superfluous and very deleterious need for ecclesiastical approbation of what it can and should do. In that respect medicine is still in the Dark Ages.

In our modern world, medicine and religion should be *completely* divorced from one another. Common sense alone will tell us that horrendous and ultimately insoluble dilemmas and crises are bound to arise and proliferate when the pressing needs of our highly sophisticated, scientific, and technological world of everyday reality are met with the wholly inadequate, inappropriate, and impotent "solutions" extracted from the miasma of so-called divine revelation, which permeated the primitive and irrelevant world of yore. It is unreasonable to expect anything but deep moral crises from the ensuing ethical sickness heralded by the resounding clash.

And those crises are now upon us. The wartime medical crimes were one result. The ethical sickness had spread to the United States even before World War II, but evidence of it surfaced only after the war, when in 1981 a horrible experiment on syphilis in Tuskegee, Alabama, was described in detail.[74] It involved a *nontherapeutic* study of 399 syphilitic black prisoners and 201 uninfected black prisoners who served as "controls." None of the subjects was asked their consent or knew what was happening.

The project began in 1932 without any organized protocol, and continued in a haphazard way until 1972—long after the Nuremberg Code had been formulated to prevent such atrocities. Some of the subjects died during this "research." Now, here was a medical crime perpetrated during times of peace and war by American doctors no more or less reputable than their German colleagues, perpetrated in the leading democratic nation whose chief justice was simultaneously (and vigorously) prosecuting those Germans for similar crimes!

What good, then, are pretentious but impotent codes? They are a charade. None of them could prevent subsequent highly unethical conduct, such as the experiment involving the injection of live cancer cells into patients without their consent or knowledge at the Sloan-Kettering Institute in New York in 1964.[75] In 1966 Dr. Henry K. Beecher at the Massachusetts General Hospital culled from the literature twenty-one instances of unethical research, sometimes involving up to 500 patients.[76] As was already mentioned in chapter 9, Pappworth cited numerous examples of unethical experimentation in his book published in 1967.[28] And in 1985, U.S. governmental documents revealed that senile and illiterate nursing home residents were unwitting "guinea pigs" for testing experimental drugs.[77] In that regard the National Council for Senior Citizens was "shocked that the very tests and practices that were forbidden years ago for prison inmates are still being conducted on senior citizens in nursing homes." A 1987 report expressed similar shock at five episodes of research in the United States using toxic doses of radioactive substances.[78] These had been done merely out of scientific curiosity on volunteers and mentally and terminally ill patients, again without their consent or knowledge.

In his analysis of the Nazi medical crimes, Dr. W. E. Seidelman of McMaster University in Hamilton, Ontario, concluded with two insightful and trenchant questions.[79] With regard to the aims, means, and circumstances of one of the most noted and previously respected German doctors, Seidelman asks: "How many of us wouldn't do the same thing? Given the *ethical vacuum in science* (italics added) . . . are we not all vulnerable?"

Ethical vacuum—that's the root of the problem. Doctors have got to come to grips with the realities of the times and fill that vacuum with a code of conduct tailored to meet the contemporary demands. And that calls for wrenching the profession entirely free of so-called *rule ethics*. According to philosopher-theologian Joseph Fletcher,[67] rule ethics mandates *a priori* what one must do "according to some predetermined precept or categorical imperative." It is a coercive, nondiscriminatory, "doctrinaire or ideological method of deciding what is right." On the other hand, *situation ethics* is a *pos-*

172 Prescription: Medicide

teriori, "relative, flexible, and changeable according to variables (from which) the moral agent, the decision maker, judges what is best in the circumstances and in the view of foreseeable consequences."

Judge Amnon Carmi of the Society for Medicine and Law in Haifa, Israel, shares this ethical stance, which ennobles human dignity by giving free reign to "the ability of man to think things over, to decide, and to apply self-control, to become his own master. . . . It is the sense of worth that comes with having the freedom and responsibility to make judgments about what is proper and improper."[80]

Fletcher anticipated the medical relevance of the situational approach, which to some physicians is simply "clinical" ethics independent of strictly moral rules. If the medical profession has any residual sense of worth, it should enthusiastically and unconditionally embrace this only workable guide to the use of reason and common sense in searching for solutions to modern ethical questions.

Those now in control of society's destiny are against my proposals simply because they cannot escape some "eternal truths" of religion or of their own rigid and unreflective opinions. They cannot distinguish rule ethics from situation (or casuistic) ethics.

One of the most powerful forces energizing the rule approach is fear of the so-called wedge or slippery slope (also known as the camel's nose under the tent, a foot in the door, and give an inch . . .) argument. All of these catchwords imply eventual moral disaster through supposedly inevitable abuse of any "radical" innovation, no matter how small or innocuous its beginning. This dread of gray zones and of imaginative novelty ultimately rests on a lack of confidence in one's ability to control—and is, in effect, an admission of character weakness.

It is absurd and degrading to offer this fear as though it were a rationally persuasive argument. That point was made by the President's Commission for the Study of Ethical Problems in Medicine, which concluded that "much more is needed than merely pointing out that allowing one kind of action (itself justified) could conceivably increase the tendency to allow another action (unjustified). Rather, it must be shown that pressures to allow the unjustified action will become so strong once the initial step is taken that the further steps are likely to occur . . . (and) such evidence is commonly quite limited."[73] Even the fear of abuse can be (and often is) abused. In its 1983 report the President's Commission warned that "slippery slope arguments are themselves subject to abuse in social and legal policy debate." If successfully foisted on society, extreme degrees of neophobia could result only in complete stagnation and ineluctable backsliding.

It is probably too much to expect—and probably too late anyway—but doctors worthy of the calling should at least try to cure their ethical infirmity by hammering out a relevant and enduring code of conduct. They must not lose sight of the fact that individually and collectively they comprise the *epitome* of medical expertise. From an idealistic point of view their opinions in medical matters cannot be superseded, and they, therefore, have the *primary* responsibility to designate what a doctor should and will do and how and when it should or will be done.

The medical profession must display the moral virility expected of that once noble calling by taking absolute control of its ethical prerogatives. The time has come—indeed is long overdue—for its leaders to create a new specialty dealing primarily with bioethics. That is a prerequisite for asserting rightful control. For the acquisition of the powers and skills needed to master the obligation, it stands to reason that it is much simpler and cheaper to train a doctor in ethics (which entails only didactics and pedagogy) than it is to train a humanist in medical art and science (which require years of didactics coupled with a tremendous amount of hands-on practice in laboratories, clinics, and operating rooms).

With that in mind I wrote an article advocating the establishment of a standard postgraduate training program (comparable to a residency) aimed at transforming certain talented, well-prepared, and strongly motivated doctors into superbly endowed bioethicists steeped in the essentials of philosophy, religion, law, and some of the arts. Tentatively called "bioethiatry" or "bioethiatrics," the new specialty would have its own board to certify bioethiatrists prepared and ready to help colleagues solve every kind of bioethical dilemma. Articles and case reports published by the new specialists in their own journal would, within a few years, form a body of rich experiences to guide legislators in the enactment of sensible statutes.

Before submitting my article to any journal, I queried a doctor associated with AMA's editorial staff about the possibilities of getting it accepted. The expected reply was quick in coming: there was absolutely no chance of acceptance. So once again I turned to the editor of the *Journal of the National Medical Association* as the only hope of having the idea exposed to at least a segment of the profession. And once again I was not disappointed.[81] This was further proof that those so-called prestigious journals are in reality not the open forums they profess to be. And the lack of any response to my article also was not unexpected.

Meanwhile, time is running out. Reverence for the traditional Hippocratic basis of medical practice is vacuous nostalgia, childish daydreaming. The profession is rapidly evolving into an integral component of the business world. If boardroom principles are not to become the ethical model for doctors, then those who dictate medical policy had better quickly take the lead in putting their ethical house in order. They are obligated to motivate every doctor to concentrate on that one point; to mobilize every resource at hand to hammer out a sensible, workable, and *timeless* code of conduct equal to the demands of our trying times and of those in the foreseeable future without the demeaning patchwork of frequent hit-or-miss revisions.

That may not be as difficult as it would appear, but only if the collective medical character is up to it. If individual doctors are properly and honestly oriented to the essence of their calling, they will need few guiding rules for their professional behavior. As Albert Einstein himself said: "When life and death are at stake, rules and obligations go by the board."[82]

The ideal doctor—the one who is always ready to do his best for any human being in real or imagined distress regardless of personality, race, life circumstances, or beliefs—doesn't exist, of course, just as the ideal human being doesn't exist. Even Hippocrates admitted that "physicians are many in title but few in reality."[72] However, doctors whose minds are free of, or can willfully be freed from, the welter of conflicting dogmatic abstractions that lead intellects in all kinds of diverse directions have the best chance of approximating the ideal.

The farthest from the ideal are doctors whose minds are, to a greater or lesser degree, so rigidly enslaved by certain beloved abstractions that only an abridged medical practice is possible for them. Their code of ethics is preordained by the source of their dogma: it doesn't matter what their patients, conventional ethics, the law, or even the deepest recesses of their oppressed minds say.

Abortion furnishes a good example of a legitimate medical service that cannot be rendered or recommended (or perhaps even thought about) by some otherwise well-trained, very competent, and dedicated practitioners. Such sheepish acquiescence by individual doctors to the artificial amputation of rational action from rational thought makes a workable consensus on bioethics impossible.

The ideal doctor, armed with a good medical education and practical training (which most doctors now have), with strong character (less commonly found), with honesty and common sense (rarer still), and with a completely free mind (rarest of all) can handle any medical challenge without having to solicit or depend upon extraneous ethical advice. But this can be true only if one essential principle remains uppermost and permanently honored in the mind of every doctor: the highest respect for the personal *autonomy or self-determination of every patient*—for what the patient deems best for his or her own earthly existence. Personal autonomy is paramount for Dr. Heyd, professor of philosophy at the Hebrew University in Jerusalem, who wrote that "the individual alone gives meaning to his life and decides whether his life is good and worth living, or not. . . . The meaning of life is a matter of decision rather than of knowledge; for in fact there is nothing to be known here. . . ."[80]

Under those conditions of patients' autonomy coupled with medical competence and honesty, how could any overwhelming or insuperable bioethical problem arise? And would an official bioethical code be at all necessary? Or even useful?

If a patient's personal creed forbids a medically indicated blood transfusion, for example, then a truly ethical doctor would not give it and would not dispute the patient's decision to refuse it. In fact, the doctor would be obligated to protest any kind of legal or judicial interference. If a patient's needs are undeniable and reasonable but require a doctor to do something illegal, then an ethically robust medical profession would fight to rescind or change the morally restrictive legislation.

When Margaret Sanger was being martyred for trying to legitimize birth control early in this century, an ethically sick medical profession didn't just stand by idly and watch; with gusto and voluntarily it helped authorities persecute and imprison her.[83] But doctors apparently didn't learn from that object lesson. They still prefer to float passively along on a hodgepodge code foisted on them by the tyranny of rule ethics applied with futility to the blind vagaries of societal evolution.

If all doctors strove to emulate the ideal with at least as much zeal as they devote to the status of their stock portfolios, if *uncompromising* benevolence had been ingrained in the medical consciousness as late as the turn of this century, then all subsequent medical controversies and crises would have remained merely incredible fantasies. Then the horrific medical war crimes would not have been committed without obvious qualms among the perpetrators and may have not been committed at all.

If *disciplined* dedication to serving any and all medical needs of humanity had been adequately evangelized, my proposal would long ago have become a reality worthy of the genuine Hippocratic spirit. And an ethically reborn guild of healers could, with unshakable confidence and entirely on its own, confront the awesome challenges sure to come in the twenty-first century.

12

The Lynching of Morality

After the populations of America's death rows began to overflow in the early 1980s, I stepped up my efforts to persuade state legislators to legitimate my proposal. Lack of money forced me to resort almost exclusively to writing letters and enclosing copies of supportive opinions from several condemned men, a few doctors, and two journalists. Only once did I indulge in the luxury of a trip for a personal appeal. In 1984, I testified before the House Committee on Jurisprudence in Austin, Texas, convened to consider an alternative sentence for those convicted of capital crimes. But I could have saved myself the price of a plane ticket; my presentation aroused no interest and no response.

Since 1981, I have contacted legislators and governors in twenty states in which an execution or some sort of official action with regard to the death penalty was pending. Whenever possible I wrote directly to the chairpersons of senate and house (or assembly) judiciary committees because they represent the source of pertinent legislation. I received replies from only four of fifty-five senators, from six of sixty-two representatives, and from four of thirty governors. Fourteen responses in all.

Most of them merely acknowledged receipt of my letter, plus the customary bland expression of gratitude for the information and an insincere promise to keep it on file. I know they were insincere, because I never heard from them about subsequent legislative developments of which I learned from other sources. A few replied that they were "not in a position to sponsor such legislation." If legislative judiciary committee members can't sponsor it, who then?

Two representatives foresaw too many logistical problems, and they felt that "the controversy engendered by such a proposal would preclude its passage at this time." My forthright and factual explanation to both of them as to how easily the logistics could be mastered, and my criticism of their reticence aroused their ire. They accused me of counterproductive stridency. I will admit to being strident, but rightfully so in the face of such moral nonchalance.

The only positive and entirely honest response came from Topeka, Kansas. In January 1987, I became aware of a bill being introduced with majority support in that state's House to reinstitute capital punishment. I telephoned the office of one of the bill's sponsors, Rep. Martha Jenkins. She had left the capital for her home in Leavenworth, but her aide assured me that the legislator would call me the following morning.

Prior experience made me skeptical of the promise. But to my surprise and delight, Rep. Jenkins called right on time. I briefly outlined my proposal and requested that the advocated choice be included in the pending legislation. She asked me to send her a written summary, and she promised to get in touch with me again. I must admit, her cordial, matter-of-fact manner did not completely dispel my lingering skepticism, especially when three weeks of silence followed.

However, on 3 February 1987 my gloomy skepticism gave way to ineffable elation on receipt of this letter:

I am sorry it has taken me so long to get back in touch with you. We were successful in passing death penalty legislation out of the full House last week. The bill (Kansas Bill 2062) contains your amendment which permits the condemned to donate their organs at the time of their execution.

Enclosed please find a copy of the amendment. The amendment is not as broad as you might have desired. It does not address the method or means by which these organ transfers are to be made.

I have been assured that the organ donation amendment will remain intact and will be a part of the bill when it becomes law.

I hope the amendment addresses your concern and offers you an opportunity to pursue legislation of this kind in other states. Thank you very much for bringing this to my attention.

How could one doubt the sincerity of that "thank you"? What an enormous, refreshing difference from other legislators.

First of all, Rep. Jenkins took immediate action—to call the bill back for amendment, without protracted and unnecessary correspondence or "analysis" of something she (and all other legislators, too) knew to be very important and timely.

Second, her dynamic response went far beyond the usual banality of the meaningless phrase, "thank you for bringing this to my attention," which tends to be the *only* response (and generally insincere, at that) from her counterparts in other states.

During the thirty-three years of my campaign, Rep. Jenkins is the only authoritative person who acknowledged, without reservation, the correctness and value of my endeavor; and she, in 1987, and Warden Ralph Alvis of Ohio in 1958 wasted no time in doing everything in their power to help make it easier for me to promote my endeavor in a morally bewildered world. They are rare individuals indeed.

The wording of the Kansas bill was general enough to authorize execution even by general anesthesia: "A person sentenced to death may make an anatomical gift in a manner and for the purposes provided by the uniform anatomical gift act and *be executed in such a manner that such a gift can be carried out* (italics added)." This represented a giant step forward, compared to the ill-fated SB 1968 proposed in Sacramento three years earlier. It not only was the first official legislative action in the United States with respect to my proposal but also incorporated the possibility of execution by general anesthesia. That broadened the scope of potential benefit far beyond the limits offered by mere lethal injection.

But I should have known that the miracle was too good to be true. A second letter came from Rep. Jenkins three months later, informing me that the bill was defeated in the Kansas Senate and the issue would not be raised again the following year.

However, another capital punishment bill was introduced in Kansas in 1989, this time in the Senate and backed by the governor. And again the Senate voted it down. Both Rep. Jenkins and the governor kept me informed of its evolution and demise. If all state officials had the same cordial and cooperative attitude, there would be no basis for bilateral rancor or for indecent and unjustifiable procrastination in pursuing the right course.

It was obvious that I still needed the help of condemned inmates if I was to make headway with state legislators. The pleas from death row would be much harder to ignore. Fortunately several condemned men in Oklahoma and Georgia agreed to become activists in my campaign. They prepared carefully worded, well-reasoned letters and concise essays, and sent them to almost all legislators in Oklahoma City and the districts around Atlanta and Macon in Georgia.

At the same time, word of all this death row activity aroused the interest of local newspaper and television journalists. Their stories assured that the matter would be taken seriously in the two capitols; indeed, some legislators responded with favorable and meaningful comments. The outlook for enabling legislation has improved and appears to be most promising in Oklahoma where lethal injection already is the official mode of execution. The use of the electric chair in Georgia presents a more formidable obstacle.

In May 1989, I sent a follow-up letter to many of those same legislators. It reinforced the inmates' pleas and clarified the technical and procedural details inherent in my proposal. As of this writing, there have been no replies.

The lack of response highlights part of the problem. Legislators are ambivalent about the relationship of law to morality. So their safest course is to do nothing, and that breeds inertia. They don't manifest a clear awareness of their role in regulating the interaction between the two concepts. And I doubt that most of them would do much about it even if they did understand or openly acknowledge the relationship.

They should know that the ultimate wellspring of morality is the mores of a people. As new conditions of life arise from the burgeoning conquests of parts of nature by science, technology, and even art, the mores adapt almost automatically. Sociologist William Sumner explained how philosophy and ethics then follow and claim to have caused the changes, which is the reverse of what really happens. Sumner concluded that "ethical notions are figments of speculation. . . . All ethics grow out of the mores and are a part of them. That is why ethics can never be antecedent to mores."[84] The late U.S. Supreme Court Justice Benjamin Cardozo also averred that "the mores are themselves variable with time and circumstance and tribe, human in origin and development. But it is out of these that . . . the 'law' has its genesis and growth."[85]

Trouble begins and grows when one tries to make laws the arbiter of morality. That was stressed by Herbert L. Packard, Professor of Law at Stanford University, who, in reference to the experience of the Prohibition era, wrote that "law, even criminal law, simply is not that potent a weapon of social control. . . . It becomes largely inefficacious when it is used to enforce morality (rather) than to deal with conduct that is generally seen as harmful."[86] And just as birth control and abortion are no longer generally seen as harmful, so, too, should the emotional stigma of taboo be stripped away from the completely moral concept of euthanasia.

It doesn't take much insight to grasp why the above rational viewpoints seem to make little, if any, impression on legislators and politicians today. Since Machiavelli's time it has been no secret that the ideas of good and evil are quite irrelevant when it comes to the acquisition and wielding of political power and influence. Einstein, too, was aware of this, and said so most pointedly: "Political leaders and governments owe their position partly to force and partly to popular election. They cannot be regarded as representative of the best elements, morally or intellectually, in their respective nations."[81] Small wonder, then, that for most politicians the genuinely valid relationship of law to morality is of little meaning or concern. They continue to ignore, or are ignorant of, what the mores are saying.

Consider birth control, for example. In the opening decades of this century the law audaciously declared the practice to be immoral and therefore illegal. However, as early as 1910 Margaret Sanger heeded the mores and recognized that birth control was moral because its time had come, no matter what the law said. In 1914 she wrote: "Shall we look upon a piece of parchment as greater than human happiness, greater than human life?"[83] Not until 1937 did misguided doctors finally come to their senses and certify birth control to be a legitimate medical service. And it took another generation before otiose lawgivers in 1973 rescinded their patently foolish and immoral laws barring its practice as a legitimate service.

The same ludicrous fracas is now being played out with regard to euthanasia. The mores are changing, and rapidly. The demand and need for controlled euthanasia and doctor-assisted suicide ripened long ago and are getting stronger. Yet utter ethical and legislative confusion and equivocation are the order of the day. Where doctors and legislators fear to tread, the judiciary has been forced to rush in and set arbitrary and haphazard precedents. The current farrago of judicial rules, regulations, penalties, and punishments desecrates human intellect and genuine morality.

More than two decades ago Chief Justice Warren Burger of the United States Supreme Court said that "in a democratic society legislatures, not courts, are constituted to respond to the will and consequently to the moral values of the people." A similar opinion was stated by Justice Felix Frankfurter in 1951: "History teaches that the independence of the judiciary is jeopardized when courts become embroiled in the passions of the day and assume primary responsibility in choosing between competing political, economic, and social pressures."[87]

Morality today is in especially grave danger from the disorganized pontifications of a hapless judiciary venturing where legislators should be. *The morality of euthanasia is being lynched by the "mob" action of courts.*

Mercy killings are on the increase. More and more doctors openly admit to having secretly helped suffering patients die.[88] Their surreptitious respect for morality seems to be echoing Margaret Sanger's courageous defiance of a half-century ago: "Shall we who respond to the throbbing pulse of human needs concern oursleves with indictments, courts, and judges, or shall we do our work first and settle with these evils after?"[83]

Evils indeed. Must death control repeat the tragic history of birth control? Must we wait another quarter of a century for an insensitive medical profession to acknowledge death control as another of its rightful responsibilities, and then wait several decades more until our somnolent law finally awakes to the call of mores?

Politicians and doctors should feel degraded for having meekly abjured their obligations in connection with euthanasia. They should feel ashamed that laypersons are being compelled to spearhead the campaign to legitimize a controlled program of planned death. Every public poll endorses the concept of euthanasia under medical control. Fifty-five percent of respondents in a poll conducted by Washington State University in May 1990 said it should be legal for a terminally ill patient to ask that a doctor hasten his or her death with sleeping pills or by injection. A coincident Times Mirror Center poll showed that an identical majority endorsed the right of an incurably ill patient to commit suicide. Even stronger support for that option came from 63 percent of responses to a 1990 Roper poll.

The trend continued and indeed increased after Janet Adkins's death. Sixty-five percent of those polled in June 1990 by *USA Today* agreed that the terminally ill should be granted medical help to end their lives. Legalization of assisted suicide was advocated by an overwhelming margin of three to one in a poll conducted by *The Flint*

(*Michigan*) *Journal* on June 24, 1990. Four days earlier *The United Methodist Reporter* (published in Dallas, Texas) revealed that 73 percent of its readers believe that it is morally justified for an individual to commit suicide under some circumstances, and 70 percent endorsed the use of assistive devices to accomplish it. Of those responding to a February 1991 poll by *Longevity* magazine, published in its June issue, fully 86 percent answered yes (11 percent said no) when asked: "Is it ever proper for a doctor to assist a patient in committing suicide?" The same percentage response was recorded for this important question: "Do you think there should be a public policy in this country to assist people who want to die?" When asked "Is it ever proper for a doctor to assist a patient in committing suicide, if the person may be years from death and not yet physically suffering greatly?" 57 percent said yes, 26 percent said no, and 17 percent didn't know.

Finally, what especially gratified me and shocked self-assured medical authorities was the (for them) unexpected solid endorsement of euthanasia and physician-assisted suicide by forty-five percent of doctors throughout the United States according to a poll published by the *Medical Tribune* on September 20, 1990. Who can doubt that the mores are speaking—indeed shouting?

Truly moral legislators and doctors would say, "*This* is to be the law, and it's simple: euthanasia is a medical service to be performed only by a duly licensed medical doctor within certain prescribed limits, like any other medical service. Only *that* is legal."

And only that is moral. It is up to the medical profession to work out the technical and procedural details, just as it does with every other facet of its complex art and science. And it should not be forgotten that the new medical service must also be available to condemned criminals because arbitrarily selective euthanasia is as immoral as no euthanasia at all.

The time is not far off when the culling of medical benefit, too, from rationally planned death will denote the highest degree of morality applied to the legal and purposeful termination of individual human lives.

13

Killing in the Shadowy Valley

It seems almost self-evident today that death is the arch enemy of medicine, to be resisted incessantly with every weapon in its arsenal. Doctors justify this implacable enmity on the basis of the Hippocratic Oath, specifically on its stipulation that they keep their patients from harm and injustice. But that is an erroneous basis.

The real source of their misconstrued primary obligation lies not in the oath but in Section II of the Second Constitution of Hippocrates' treatise on epidemics.[72] Physicians are exhorted by the father of their calling "to do good *or* to do no harm" (italics added). A doctor's art entails the constellation of the disease, the patient, and himself; the doctor and his patient are to work together *to combat the disease.* Nowhere is it stated that the doctor must heroically lead his patient off to do battle with death.

It is clear that as far as Hippocrates was concerned the main, indeed the *only,* enemy is disease—that is, the disturber of a person's "ease." And the means to fight that enemy is the art of medicine, the *servant* of which is the doctor (who today has instead made himself its lord). In having taken the tack of combating death, in thus having usurped a prerogative never advanced by its revered progenitor, the medical profession wantonly infringes both aspects of its special and genuinely Hippocratic obligation: In quixotically trying to conquer death, doctors all too frequently do no good for their patients' "ease"; but, at the same time, they do harm instead by prolonging and even magnifying patients' dis-ease.

This monomaniacal and ultimately foolish obsession with subduing death is one side of the same coin. The other side is medicine's equally misguided commitment to maintaining life at all costs (which comprises a fairly large chunk of our gross national product). This contrived obligation serves as the basis of an implied commandment for doctors not to purposely kill any human being, and therefore to reject euthanasia or mercy killing.

As another "official and incontrovertible" justification for that commandment, doctors point to this short sentence in the oath: "I will neither give a deadly drug to anybody if asked for it, nor will I make a suggestion to this effect."[64] Therefore, for them euthanasia is absolutely unethical. This may be true for a good number of today's doctors, but it wasn't always so, not even in Hippocrates' day. Besides, their unjust stand against euthanasia also rests on a faulty interpretation of the real meaning of that sentence in the oath.

According to historian Ludwig Edelstein, whose analysis of the oath is considered to be the most authoritative, suicide was common in antiquity and not disgraceful if there was a good reason for it. The only opposition came from the Pythagoreans, who outlawed suicide unconditionally as a sin against their gods, and that inflexible stand carried over into Christian dogma.

The commonest means for suicide back then was poison. Patients knew that doctors possessed the means for an easy and painless death and were likely to demand that doctors give them the drugs for that purpose. Edelstein emphasizes that such demands were not made or taken lightly. A patient wracked with mental or physical stress usually consulted a doctor to decide whether treatment was worth continuing. If the doctor judged the outlook hopeless, then directly or indirectly he suggested suicide.

Edelstein concludes that euthanasia was an everyday occurrence in those times—something which all interpreters of the oath overlook or ignore. And, he adds, "it is the neglect of the question of euthanasia that gave currency to the belief that in the Oath not only suicide but also manslaughter are forbidden. . . . It suffices here to state that in antiquity many physicians actually gave their patients the poison for which they were asked."[64]

Hopelessly tied to a misinterpretation of the oath, a misguided medical profession has for centuries been responsible for much unnecessary suffering and personal degradation by refusing to hasten a merciful death for pleading patients. To me it is incredible that a doctor could abide the agony of a doomed human simply because of a personal commitment to an invented abstraction, be it mere opinion or some exalted principle born of cogitation. As philosopher Samuel Gorowitz states, the price of a doctor steadfastly adhering to his own personal convictions in refusing to aid or perform euthanasia is not extracted from his or her own life, but is thereby imposed on the suffering patient who professes a different set of values. "Thus," chides Gorowitz, "(the doctor) becomes one whose values demand behavior that results in the impoverishment in the lives of others, and which therefore will be seen by many to be parochial, inhumane, and unjustified."[89]

How unwittingly cruel for doctors in various nations throughout history to have stood by idly while thousands were being brutally crucified, crushed, and burned to death; while "heretics" like their own colleague, Dr. Michael Servetus, were being cooked alive at the stake, and others ripped to pieces during the Middle Ages. Our own time is no different: men and women are being gassed, hanged, and "comfortably fried" sitting down.

Why didn't the powerful medical profession rise up as a whole and scream, "No! Let *us* do it humanely. Let us kill him with an opiate"? Why doesn't the profession rise up now and *demand* the same for all doomed humans today? Why do doctors continue to

ignore the rare example of Drs. Guillotin and Louis? Their contribution, though unintentionally gory, nonetheless manifested at least
an awareness of the compassion expected from a supposedly benevolent profession apparently unwilling or unable to discern the crucial
difference between strident compassion and gushing sentimentality.
It's high time doctors showed some "tough love."

Euthanasia wasn't of much interest to me until my internship
year, when I saw first-hand how cancer can ravage the human body.
The patient was a helplessly immobile woman of middle age, her entire
body jaundiced to an intense yellow-brown, skin stretched paper-thin
over a fluid-filled abdomen swollen to four or five times normal size.
The rest of her was an emaciated skeleton: sagging, discolored skin
covered her bones like a cheap, wrinkled frock.

The poor wretch stared up at me with yellow eyeballs sunken
in their atrophic* sockets. Her yellow teeth were ringed by chapping
and parched lips to form an involuntary, almost sardonic "smile"
of death. It seemed as though she was pleading for help and death
at the same time. Out of sheer empathy alone I could have helped
her die with satisfaction. From that moment on, I was sure that doctor-
assisted euthanasia and suicide are and always were ethical, no matter
what anyone says or thinks.

But that was true long before I became aware of it. While on
a steamship trip to New York in April 1910, Mark Twain was suffering such intense pain and discomfort from chronic heart disease that
he pleaded with his business partner to kill him and end his misery.[90]
Others who were and are famous and have access to the means either
do it themselves or secretly get help from their doctors. In the
seventeenth century the noted Dr. William Harvey died at the age
of eighty "it is said from the effects of opium which he had taken
with suicidal intent to escape the suffering from painful gout."[91] In
our own century, that paragon of sanity Dr. Sigmund Freud submitted
to thirty-three operations for cancer of the jaw and endured sixteen
years of terrible pain before he had his personal doctor carry out

---

*Withering

a prior agreement to end his suffering through comatose death induced by two doses of morphine.[92] In 1936 the British royal family approved the clandestine euthanasia of King George V who was dying of "bronchial catarrh and left-sided heart weakness." His personal doctor injected lethal doses of morphine and cocaine to shorten the final stage of agony and thereby avert a death, as the doctor put it, "without the dignity and serenity which he most richly deserved."[93]

Now, I am not aware of any official denunciation of the doctors involved in the above examples as having been unethical. If, therefore, such conduct was ethical then, it's ethical now. Why the obvious double standard? What is good enough for the *aristoi* is also good enough for the *hoi polloi*. *Common people, too, must not be forced to die without the dignity and serenity which they also most richly deserve.*

An epochal breakthrough in this regard is taking place today in the Netherlands where euthanasia, although technically illegal, is openly tolerated and practiced within unofficial but very strict guidelines sanctioned by court decisions. Taking advantage of that refreshing leniency, about one doctor out of every five among the 120,000 members of the Dutch medical profession openly performs euthanasia.[94] In this way they end the agony of almost 10,000 patients every year.

I first learned of that remarkable triumph of common sense in 1986. Then I conceived the idea of expanding my death row proposal to include experimentation on willing patients who opt for euthanasia. And because I mistakenly assumed that the practice was legal there, the Netherlands seemed to be the logical place to try to implement the idea.

Arriving in Amsterdam in the summer of 1987, my first stop was at the office of the Society for Voluntary Euthanasia. During the following week I had several long conversations with the director. It was a bit disheartening to learn that euthanasia was still illegal there and that the national legislature was reluctant to give it official legitimacy. That bit of overt hypocrisy was annoying, to say the least.

Another less unexpected disappointment was the vague but discernible negative reaction to my long-range aim of terminal experimentation. The director expressed concern that my idea would be so radical an innovation that mere debate about it would halt, or even set back, the long, hard struggle to win public acceptance for simply putting a suffering patient to death. I appreciated that concern, and had concluded on my own that the official illegality of euthanasia dashed all hope of achieving what I had planned. But I was interested in what two noted Dutch euthanasists might say about my plan. I made arrangements to meet with anesthesiologist Dr. Pieter V. Admiraal in Delft and with general practitioner Dr. Herbert Cohen near Rotterdam.

Dr. Admiraal received me in his office in a modern suburban hospital about thirty-five miles southwest of Amsterdam. I was immediately impressed by his calm, down-to-earth manner and an unmistakable aura of competence and integrity. He told me that he performed euthanasia only in cases of terminal cancer, which up to that time numbered over one hundred. When I asked what he thought of my advocacy of experimentation on willing patients opting for euthanasia, and how it might be received by Dutch authorities, his curt reply amused me: "They'd hang you!" he said without hesitation.

It was Dr. Admiraal who drew up the guidelines now accepted by Dutch judicial authorities as the proper way to perform euthanasia.[94] Briefly, they stipulate that an unbearably agonized patient must express a firm, voluntary, and unwavering wish to die, even when fully informed about other potential forms of therapy and about possible clinical courses. The decision to proceed must involve more than one professional person, and a doctor must be included to insure competency in the choice and use of drugs. Finally, and most astonishingly, the procedure is available not only to the terminally ill, but also to others suffering from crippling paraplegia, arthritis, multiple sclerosis, and even chronic bronchitis.[95]

I had the pleasure of relaxed conversation with Dr. Cohen while enjoying a dinner at an outdoor restaurant overlooking a marina in Rotterdam. He told me that he performed an average of one euthanasia per month, using an injected barbiturate to induce unconsciousness followed by a muscle paralyzer to cause death within several minutes. He followed the set guidelines and insisted on repeated consultations before acting.

Relatives of patients are not involved in the decision process. As Cohen put it: "First, it's none of their business. You have to respect the patient's autonomy. Second, a relative involved in making a decision might feel guilty afterward."[94] Even at the last moment Cohen asks if patients really wouldn't want to live a while longer, and they usually decline in the strongest terms.

In Cohen's opinion there is no difference between helping a patient commit suicide and actually performing euthanasia. He has done both. But in the United States there is a legal difference. However, American law is slipshod and murky, and just as chaotic as medical ethics with regard to euthanasia.

Depending on the state or political entity and the law enforcement personalities involved, a doctor who performs euthanasia in the United States faces a spectrum of unpredictable penalties, ranging from none at all, through suspended sentence, probation, limited incarceration, life imprisonment, and—theoretically only—a death sentence. Of course, the charge of murder is absurd, as the legal definition in chapter 11 makes abundantly clear. Under current state laws the only admissible charge for having committed active euthanasia would be voluntary manslaughter, meaning the actual performance of the willful and unlawful killing of a human being without malice, either express or implied[65] (in contrast to the passive euthanasia of merely letting die). These crazy-quilt legal distinctions in America make it dangerous and even deadly for some doctors to do what they know is right.

The tragic case of Dr. John Kraai is a good example. In 1985 the seventy-six-year-old general practitioner in a town near Rochester, New York, was charged with second degree murder for having injected a lethal dose of insulin into his eighty-one-year-old nursing home patient suffering from Alzheimer's disease and gangrene of the feet.[96] The old man had been Kraai's patient for over forty years. Many of the doctor's other patients rallied to his support. To their dismay he was found dead shortly afterwards, apparently due to a self-injected drug. The president of the local county medical society lamented the "sorry end to a long career of service for a man who spent his entire life taking care of people." But it should not be forgotten that Kraai's own profession was indirectly responsible for that sorry end.

Back in Michigan and inspired by my visit to the Netherlands, I decided to take the risky step of assisting terminal patients in committing suicide. I could not even consider performing active euthanasia and thereby being charged with murder in a very hostile milieu. Merely helping with self-killing would entail less risk. It would also help clarify the law.

The legal befuddlement is there for all to see. Fortunately, the old common law condemnation of suicide as a crime has been rescinded. Suicide, attempted or successful, is no longer a criminal act. How, then, can *assisting* someone to perform that legal act be called criminal and illegal? But that sort of blatant irrationality is incorporated into the laws of at least thirty of our states, and therefore makes assisted suicide a risky action, too. When word of my plans reached the county prosecutor's office, I was threatened with the possible charge of first degree murder (of all things!) if I helped patients die—despite my protest that aiding a suicide can never be murder.

My view that assisting in a suicide is not murder was based on a recent case in Michigan.[97] It involved two young men, Steven Campbell and Kevin Basnaw, who had been drinking heavily one night in 1980. When Basnaw announced that he intended to kill himself, Campbell went home and returned with his own handgun and five bullets, which he placed on a table in front of Basnaw. Campbell then departed. Basnaw was found the next morning slumped over the table, gun in hand. Campbell was charged in St. Clair County Circuit Court with open murder.*

Justification for the charge of murder stemmed from a 1920 Michigan case in which a thirty-six-year-old man named Roberts was convicted of murder for having placed a potion of poison within the reach of his terminally ill wife at her request. He was sentenced to life imprisonment without parole, at hard labor, and in solitary confinement! However, that outrage was ameliorated the same year when

---

*The degree has not yet been specified but the actual charge is pending.

his sentence was reduced to five years; he was later released from prison after three years.[97]

The appellate judges who reviewed the Campbell case reversed the trial court's warrant and discharged him in 1983. The judges explained that "the (1920) decision does not represent the law of Michigan. The term suicide excludes by definition homicide. Simply put, the defendant here did not kill another person. . . . Incitement to suicide has not been held to be a crime in two-thirds of the states . . . (and) *where incitement to suicide has been held to be a crime, there has been no unanimity as to the nature or severity of the crime. . . . What constitutes the crime of incitement to suicide is vague and undefined, and no reasonably ascertainable standard of guilt has been set forth. . . . The remedy for this situation is in the legislature*" (italics added).[97]

Consequently, the prosecutor's empty threat could not deter me, because in the final analysis I would not be inciting suicide. In fact, like the Dutch euthanasists, I would even try talking patients out of taking their own lives, and then assist them only as a last resort.

The first step was to decide on the method I was to use. Supplying drugs for the patient to swallow would be too much like active euthanasia. Then I recalled that in our medical school lectures on pathology the professor somewhat cynically remarked that carbon monoxide offers the best way to commit suicide. The pure gas has no color, taste, or smell; and it's toxic enough to cause rapid unconsciousness in relatively low concentration. Furthermore, in light complexioned people it often produces a rosy color that makes the victim look better as a corpse.

Therefore, I intended to advise patients and their families on where to obtain the gas and how it was to be administered under my supervision. A thin plastic tube would connect a small gas canister or tank to a routine plastic mask over the patient's nose and mouth, as routinely done in hospitals for oxygen therapy. I would attach ECG electrodes to the patient to monitor heart action. The gas would be turned on by the patient at a time of his or her choosing, with the rate of flow previously adjusted to cause death in about five minutes—to be verified by the ECG tracing.

But theory is one thing, reality another. I knew that there was no hope of using medical journals to let medical colleagues in the immediate area know of the existence of this new and unique service. However, the editor of a weekly medical newspaper in Detroit was interested in the idea and published a comprehensive article about it entitled "Death by Appointment: Medical Management of Death."[99] It, too, failed to evince any response from doctors or patients.

Most of the terminal patients who might want to make use of the service are under the care of cancer specialists called oncologists. My next step, then, was to make personal contact with as many oncologists as possible, almost all of whom were strangers to me. To facilitate and formalize introductions, I had business cards printed with my name, followed by the name of my new practice: "Bioethics and obitiatry. Special death counseling, by appointment only." There was also a blank line for me to write in my phone number. To add a touch of dignity and legitimacy to the new specialty, I coined the word "obitiatry," the meaning of which will be explained shortly.

I was now ready to find out if oncologists were willing to cooperate. Some of them were on staff at university-affiliated hospitals. But every one of them refused to cooperate in even the most indirect or remote way. A few were sincerely and steadfastly opposed to euthanasia, but in most instances abstention was due to fear of criminal prosecution.

It wasn't their refusal per se that dismayed me, but their unfounded fear—unfounded because there could be no question of complicity if patients were merely informed and left to contact me on their own, without any sort of referral by their doctors. And deplorable because, during discussions, at least half of the oncologists privately endorsed what I planned to do and verified the need for it in their own practices.

Another dismaying experience awaited me when a fair-minded oncologist arranged for me to meet with assistants and a few staff members of his department at a university-affiliated hospital near Detroit. The group consisted mainly of nurses, a few medical students and technologists, and three doctors. They listened to my presentation with interest. There were few outright responses, but a couple of positive ones came from nurses. Word of the meeting reached hospital authorities, who promptly cancelled a second session (for all the doctors in the department) scheduled for a few days later. That was in 1987, and the hospital's ban is still in effect in 1991, even though doctor-assisted suicide has begun to receive cautious ethical imprimatur as evidenced by a recently published journal article.[88,100]

With the refusal of oncologists to help, I knew that I would somehow have to advertise the availability of the option. Therefore, I placed a small ad for several weekdays and a weekend in the classified "Professional Services" section of a local newspaper and in the "Medical/Dental Counseling" section of a major Detroit daily (see figure 3). Again, no meaningful response.

Maybe the ads were too unobtrusive. Maybe they were taken to be a charlatan's macabre get-rich-quick scheme or merely the prank of a "kook." Only two persons called. One was a distraught man whose brother had been in coma for more than six months in another state. I explained to the pleading man that I could not help his brother, because he was not mentally competent and also because he was in another state where the procedure is illegal. The second respondent was a young woman whose rambling talk about a relative indicated mental instability, and I quickly and discreetly ended the conversation.

Up to this point I have considered euthanasia only in connection with condemned criminals and hopelessly ill or incapacitated patients. But as a merciful option it should also be available to others inextricably trapped in circumstances mandating certain death. I have arbitrarily categorized the circumstances as follows:

Obligatory Assisted Suicide

This includes everyone who must, without exception or recourse, be put to death by a person or agency having sole jurisdiction over the killing. Obviously only those condemned to some form of official or unofficial execution, not necessarily judicial, are in this group. The victims may or may not be criminals per se, and the executioners

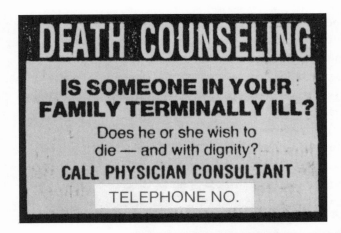

Figure 3. My classified newspaper ads, placed in June 1987

may or may not be legitimately empowered—for example, the purge of politicians during and after revolutions, gangland-style executions, and even some random murders.

Optional Assisted Suicide

This is for those individuals, sometimes in good physical and mental health, who choose to be killed by another as the preferable of only two almost equally unpleasant alternatives. Included are individuals who decide that they must die because of absolutely invincible factors, but who for some reason cannot kill themselves.

The compelling factors may be physical (the end stage of incurable disease, crippling deformity, or severe trauma), mental (intense anxiety or psychic torture inflicted by self or others), or doxastic (religious or philosophic tenets or inflexible personal convictions). Also in this group would be the forebears of Christianity in ancient Rome, whose "choice" to be killed by hungry lions in the Coliseum was preferable to the alternative "choice" of renouncing their faith (spiritual death).

The martyrs of Masada in the first century A.D. also fall into this group. Hopelessly besieged by Roman legions, all but one of the almost one thousand Jewish Zealots committed optional assisted suicide. Using swords and knives, fathers "gave freedom" to their children; husbands to their wives; bachelors to fathers and husbands; and the ten leaders to the bachelors. The last Zealot killed himself by falling on his shortened javelin. However, the shaft broke under his weight, leaving him propped up on his knees and bleeding profusely. The shaft then slipped in the blood, and he fell flat, screaming in pain. He pleaded for one of the five women, designated to hide and survive, to get a knife and end his misery. But he died anyway, whispering, "A last command—kill me! The pain gets between me and God. Kill me. Life is a . . . calamity."[101]

Could there be a more eloquent and persuasive argument for euthanasia?

Obligatory Suicide

This category comprises those irrevocably condemned to kill themselves. Here a combination of extrinsic and intrinsic pressure forces the self-destruction exemplified by the last Zealot. A more current example is the Japanese ritual of *hara-kiri* (literally, "stomach cutting"). Only by performing this solemn but gruesome act can a devout Shintoist guilty of intolerable sin gain "passage into the next life."

The highly stylized ritual calls for the piercing of the left upper abdomen with a ten-inch sword and, without showing any emotion, gradually sweeping it across to the right side, ending with a slight upward cut. In the seventeenth century the act was embellished by the Samurai code of *seppuku*: hara-kiri with simultaneous beheading by sword, the latter being carried out by the victim's best friend to minimize suffering.[102] Today these rituals are officially discouraged and frowned upon in Japan but are still generally regarded as honorable, and even occasionally performed.

The ritual suicide of *suttee* in India also fits this category. It requires a widow to immolate herself on the funeral pyre cremating her dead husband. The practice has been vehemently denounced by the Indian government, but rare instances still occur among peasants in poor rural areas.

If these examples seem too remote and exotic, then consider another one closer in time and space, and involving healthy Americans. It ranks as one of the most bizarre episodes of obligatory suicide in modern times: the mass death by cyanide of almost one thousand fanatic adherents of the Jim Jones religious cult in Guyana in 1978. Diehard critics of euthanasia would probably argue that the awful scene of many contorted bodies of men, women, and children scattered willy-nilly over the shrubby fields was less grotesque than would be the imagined scene of the same bodies handled in an individual and respectfully proper way after an even more serene death in an orderly clinical setting.

Optional Suicide

For persons who are in no way afflicted by illness but who have arbitrarily and irrevocably decided that they must die, it is well known that a number sometimes condemn themselves for no objective reason. Psychiatrists suspect that hereditary as well as environmental factors play a part, but nobody really knows why and how that is so. The incidence of such suicides is rising, especially rapidly among the elderly who manifested a 25 percent increase during the first half of the 1980s. According to geriatrician Dr. Robert Butler, "there's a much greater awareness of . . . incurable disease, and people know they're going to become helpless and the costs are going to be great."[103]

Historically, all efforts at preventing suicide have had little success. Around the seventh century the authorities tried to discourage it by declaring the act to be "sinful"; three centuries later, "immoral"; then around 1350, "illegal." In the seventeenth century those who committed suicide were declared to have been insane, their property was confiscated, their families condemned, and their corpses desecrated by ignominious burial or "insulted" by mutilation or by having horses defecate on them.[103,104] But suicides continued unabated.

Today there is an almost irresistible tendency to look for some sort of mental illness as the ultimate cause in every case of self-induced death, perhaps triggered by an episode of depression. Obviously this doesn't apply in instances of daring individuals, such as soldiers, killing themselves in reckless acts of bravery. Psychiatrists might explain this type of benevolent self-sacrifice as the satisfaction of a moot death wish.

On the other hand, some suicidologists acknowledge a distinction between "rational" and "irrational" suicide. Distinguished professor of law Glanville Williams doubts whether a suicide attempt necessarily indicates mental illness or justification for commitment for psychiatric therapy.[104] And Judge Amnon Carmi cites other authorities who maintain that suicide is not necessarily a desperate or evil act by reason of insanity, and that a man's life and death are equally his own.[80] Therefore, someone who intervenes to prevent a suicide on the basis of his or her own opinion or personal worldview runs the risk of unduly infringing the personal autonomy of a rational subject, no matter how well intentioned the intervention. And I agree with Williams's contention that we sometimes continue to endure otherwise intolerable adversity only *because* of the option of suicide as an escape, which comforts us enough so that the felt need to exercise the option is dissipated or ameliorated.

I am convinced that the mere availability of euthanasia and physician-assisted suicide will avert the panic known to motivate many apparently senseless suicides. Furthermore, it is conceivable that in the future the accumulated experience of many years underlying a well-established, tightly controlled, and finely honed program of euthanasia will afford a reliable and objective gauge for distinguishing potentially irrational suicide. After all, would anyone in his or her right mind prefer to contemplate self-destruction with other conventional and certainly less pleasant means, and under less than optimal circumstances?

Suicide by Proxy

This category encompasses the killing, by the decision and action of another, of fetuses, infants, minor children, and every human being incapable of giving direct or informed consent. Abortions and the killing of anencephalic infants are current examples of this group; although still controversial, especially in the case of the latter, the act in both instances is generally deemed to be ethical.

The situation with regard to the other individuals listed is still being hotly debated among bioethicists, legislators, and the general public, and is beyond the scope of this book. Its eventual legal status will be determined by the outcome of very emotional debates over so-called right-to-die bills now being introduced in many state legislatures. (There is no such thing as a "right" to die, but rather only a right to choose when or how to die.)

But the legal status, whatever it turns out to be, will not determine the true morality of action associated with individuals in this category. That is the primary obligation of the medical profession, no matter how soul-wrenching and disagreeable. And until doctors tackle the problem vigorously and with unshackled ratiocination, the validity of moral judgment as well as the law here will always be in doubt.

The above list of categories encompasses all potential candidates for the humane killing known as euthanasia, by others or by self. But merciful or not, sanctioned or not, such a death is always negative in our everyday world. It is ultimately a loss—the loss of life— and by definition that is the negativity of detraction. So, euthanasia is and always has been a purely negative concept, no matter how it's done or what qualifying label is put on it. I am trying to persuade society to turn it around into something positive. I believe that death in every category discussed can be merciful and at the same time yield something of real value to the suffering humanity left behind.

The medical profession's single-minded obsession with the longevity of life has blinded it to other special needs of society and has spawned the inevitable ethical dilemmas now upon us. Rapidly changing socioeconomic and demographic conditions will soon force the intransigent medical profession to accept planned death by euthanasia, even if only of the negative kind. Then the profession would be doing the right thing, but for the wrong reason: it would have acted only because it was forced to do so.

The right thing and the right reason for doing it were advocated in France back in 1919, but fell on deaf ears throughout the world. Perhaps only because the need for it then wasn't plain for all to see, nobody took seriously Dr. Binet-Sangle's farsighted proposal for the establishment of professionally staffed and well-equipped "suicide centers" for the sole purpose of assuring a humane and painless death for all those who need and desire it.[106] The time has come not only to consider his idea but to make the "quantum leap" of supplementing merciful killing with the enormously positive benefit of experimentation and organ donation.

Surgeons who now exploit brain-dead patients for those purposes are vulnerable to justifiable criticism because of their *primary* aim in behaving that way. What they really want is to get the organs or to get a chance for some kind of risky research otherwise impossible to do on humans (such as the unpublicized artificial heart implants mentioned in chapter 11). They are not concerned first and foremost with assuring the best possible death for the brain-dead patients, or even with doing everything in their power to keep them alive in that comatose state (which is what they say their oath tells them to do).

The errant surgeons rationalize their self-serving conduct as being in the interest of their patients, but by that they mean in the interest of their recipient patients first, not of the brain-dead patients who have priority in the dispensation of care as long as life remains in their bodies. In this way the surgeons' "abhorrence" of euthanasia compels them to misguided infringement of one of their most cited Hippocratic maxims. As already mentioned, they compound the infringement by neglecting to use anesthesia during the removal of organs from the brain-dead patients, thereby subjecting them to the unknown and unknowable risk of potentially excruciating and absolutely undetectable pain.

The same is true in how doctors handle the killing of fetuses. They now take pancreatic tissue from live and aborted fetuses for implantation into diabetic patients. Adults suffering from Parkinson's disease ("shaking palsy") are receiving transplants of fetal brain tissue. Despite a raging debate, organs are being taken from live anencephalic infants. Furthermore, sometimes grisly experiments are being performed on aborted fetuses, such as the one in Finland funded by the U. S. Department of Health, Education, and Welfare in the early 1970s, wherein the severed heads of fetuses were kept "alive" by being attached to a blood-oxygenator.[107] Researchers are also contemplating *in utero* experiments on live fetuses scheduled to be aborted.[108]

This disjointed research activity at the fringes of law and morality could be centralized, rationally organized, well controlled, and ethically validated in official "suicide centers" created specifically for the good of moribund subjects by affording them a serene, dignified death as well as a proper atmosphere for completely ethical manipulations. The latter objectives, such as getting their organs and doing experiments on them, would then be above reproach. They would be entirely ethical spinoffs of the main aim if pursued within well-reasoned and solidly inculcated guidelines (see the Appendix) and sensible legislation. This open and formal approach would also minimize the probability of abuse.

It should be obvious that the envisioned innovative by-products of mercy killing call for new terms to distinguish them from what is traditionally known as euthanasia, which now is not the simple concept it once was. Therefore, I propose that the term "euthanasia" be restricted to denote the termination of life performed by anybody. If performed only by professional medical personnel (such as a doctor, nurse, paramedic, physician's assistant, or medical technologist), then it becomes *medicide.*

Such a unique "suicide center" as described above obviously would offer society more than empty, negative death. Its much more important *positive* mission calls for a name worthy of that noble purpose. Because "suicide" and "euthanasia" have ineradicably negative connotations, I coined the word *obitorium* (from the Latin *obitus*, meaning "to go to meet death") for the center, and *obitiatry* (pronounced oh-bit-eye-a-tree, and using *iatros* meaning "doctor" in Greek) for the specialty. Logically its practitioner would then be an obitiatrist.

Therefore, obitiatry is the name of the medical specialty concerned with the treatment or doctoring of death to achieve some sort of beneficial result, in the same way that psychiatry is the name of the medical specialty concerned with the treatment or doctoring of the psyche for the beneficial result of mental health. In other words, medicide is euthanasia, but euthanasia may not be medicide. And obitiatry is medicide, but medicide may not be obitiatry.

The time has come to let medicide extend a comforting hand to those slipping into the valley of death, and to let obitiatry extract from their ebbing vitality the power to illuminate some of its darkest recesses for those who come after them.

14

The Quality of Mercy Unstrained

The proclamation by a special medical panel in March 1989 that it is ethical for doctors to help terminal patients commit suicide was a milestone breakthrough for me.[100] This unexpected development reinforced my determination to meet a pressing need by once again openly offering the option of assisted self-euthanasia as a professional service.

The special panel consisted of twelve prominent doctors convened by the Society for the Right to Die, based in New York City. Their report stated: "All but two of us believe that it is not immoral for a physician to assist in the rational suicide of a terminally ill person." The two dissenters eventually joined in to make the announced decision unanimous.[100]

When I learned of the panel's sudden enlightenment, I wrote a letter to its chairman and to the editors of two "prestigious" medical journals. Mincing no words, I rebuked them and the profession for having so long delayed endorsing a concept they well knew was ethical but about which they had remained silent. I was angry because doctors continued to snub my unique and perhaps newly created medical practice, which, in the end, they meekly and reluctantly are beginning to admit is legitimate. I was angry because my audacious activity in that regard, without precedent in the United States, still could not shake the medical profession out of its torpor concerning euthanasia. My anger remained because even supportive doctors were paralyzed by the fear of recrimination, censure, stigmatization, and disgrace. This includes the distinguished panel members. They shied away from endorsing outright what a sixth of the Dutch medical profession has been doing humanely and competently for years—namely, active euthanasia performed by doctors themselves.

With the panel's announcement the American Medical Association suddenly appeared interested by ostensibly committing its journal to an open debate on euthanasia. With the publication of a safely "anonymous" confession entitled "It's Over, Debbie"[109] by a doctor who supposedly committed euthanasia on a comatose patient without consent, the AMA tried—much too late and too ineptly—to pretend that it had been a champion of, or at least sympathetic to, free dialogue all along.

On the contrary, the AMA's ploy merely acknowledged that it could no longer resist the pressures of social evolution. These pressures reflect the burgeoning demand for the acceptance and use of euthanasia as practiced in the Netherlands. Even in several other countries where active euthanasia is illegal, such as Switzerland, the former West Germany, and Uruguay, doctors are not prosecuted if they adhere to certain guidelines in assisting the suicide of consenting patients who are imminently terminal. Like it or not, the AMA now *has* to begin participating openly in the trend, but as a follower, not as a leader. This should not surprise anyone familiar with the AMA's regrettable history in connection with past social innovations. It has assumed the posture of wanton self-service. Organized medicine bitterly opposed many socially progressive steps that it feared might unravel its lucrative monoply.

A few examples prove it. In the late nineteenth century the AMA opposed the idea of women becoming doctors. It issued this outlandish argument: "When a critical case demands independent action and fearless judgment, man's success depends on his virile courage, which the normal woman does not have nor is expected to have."[18] Yet it was Margaret Sanger, a *nurse* with boundless courage, who in the next century weathered the vicious persecution of those "virile" men and forced them to grudgingly admit they were wrong.

Continuing its deplorable behavior, the AMA declared it to be unethical for any doctor to be involved with any kind of group practice or salaried employment. In the 1930s the AMA stubbornly opposed the establishment of health insurance plans and fought against Medicare in the mid-1960s with unspeakable ferocity. All of these "threatening" changes proved to be absolutely indispensable for the survival of modern medical practice and are now unarguably ethical and gratefully championed by their former, albeit unrepentant, foe.

So, how can it be doubted that the AMA's "Debbie" farce is the first step in another impending social flip-flop? I predict that within a decade or two the AMA will strive to cultivate the image of having ennobled the guild it represents through "bold" leadership in the acceptance of euthanasia. It will do so in the hope, of course, that the public will have forgotten its prior blind and senseless opposition to the concept.

The special panel recommended that medical assistance be limited to the prescribing and ordering of a lethal dose of a drug to be swallowed by the patient. On resuming my efforts, I still planned to use carbon monoxide. However, several nagging doubts remained. First, there is the unavoidable risk (small though it may be) of harm to others in the immediate area as a result of an accident or of faulty use of the gas. Second, some patients, especially those prone to claustrophobia, might suffer discomfort or stress in having to breathe through a plastic mask placed over the nose and mouth. Third, the patient may be incapable of exerting enough force, or even enough movement, to turn a valve. Fourth, popularization of the procedure and the general availability of canisters of the gas could lead to wholesale "copycat" suicides by others who are in no way terminally or physically ill. That in turn could evoke such a powerful emotional reaction from various clerical and lay factions as to force the voluntary or legal curtailment of supplies of carbon monoxide for that purpose.

In addition, there are nagging doubts about the panel's envisioned method. A barbiturate would seem to be what they had in mind. Cyanide kills more quickly, but as discussed earlier, in a way not much different from suffocation. Barbiturate coma undoubtedly is more humane and therefore preferable.

Then there's the question of dosage. In the case of cyanide one pill will do. A lethal dose of barbiturates requires many pills or capsules. That would make some patients gag violently, and those who would not gag might be too debilitated by illness to swallow even a single pill. If a dose taken is less than lethal, the patient may languish in deep coma for a long time, and may suffer enough drug-induced brain damage to end up in a prolonged vegetative state. Breathing and heartbeat could be so deeply depressed that it would be hard to time the occurrence of death even with an ECG.

I concluded that only a rapid, serene, and sure method would do—intravenous (I.V.) injection. Under current laws anyone who kills a patient by injection would be guilty of at least voluntary manslaughter. Therefore, the injection somehow had to be self-administered.

After some thought I hit upon a way to do it. I would perform a venipuncture on the patient and start an I.V. drip of normal saline solution. Then, at the time of the patient's choosing I would turn on a monitoring ECG as he or she pressed a hair-trigger switch to activate a special mechanism that would perform several functions. The first three would be simultaneous: stopping of the saline drip, starting a rapid infusion of a large dose of thiopental through tubing connected to the same I.V. needle, and finally triggering a timer. Sixty seconds later the timer would start a rapid infusion of concentrated potassium chloride solution to flow concurrently with the thiopental through the same I.V. needle. The timer would also have turned off the device, but the solutions would continue to flow.

As a result of this the patient would be put into deep coma

within twenty to thirty seconds by the thiopental solution, and the potassium chloride will have paralyzed the heart muscle within several minutes. In effect, then, the patient will have had a painless heart attack while in deep sleep. In all probability death will have occurred within three to six minutes after the device is activated, and cessation of heartbeat will be verified by the ECG tracing.

Cogitation about this method was the easy part. Creating the device proved to be quite a challenge, especially because I lacked access to sophisticated and very expensive machine shop tools. With several tentative designs in mind I searched lumber and hardware outlets, "flea markets," garage sales, and my own accumulated pile of useless junk for several knick-knacks that could possibly be used. These included small clock motors, parts from toys, tiny pulleys and chains, and electrical magnets and switches.

Working by the seat of my pants, without the use of drawings, and with the help of ordinary household tools (including a small electric drill and soldering iron), in late August 1989, first one, then another contraption was constructed, but neither worked. I needed a stronger clock motor, a better switch, and a more powerful solenoid. As luck would have it, I found all three at a local "flea market" for a total cost of three dollars. That completed the device's internal mechanism. Using scrap aluminum sheeting and bars I fashioned a shiny cover and an extendible handle to also serve as a stand for the I.V. solutions. Excluding labor, the total cost was about thirty dollars.

The prototype device, which I dubbed the "Mercitron" (see figure 4), was ready in early September and functioned well on repeated testing with the solutions draining into a small receptacle. But the real test would come when they drained into the vein of a biologically live subject. Almost by mental reflex one assumes that the first subject should be an animal. And what would be more appropriate than a stray dog that must be "put to sleep" in a pound? Again, easier said than done.

Naively disregarding potential bureaucratic obstacles, I requested permission to try the device on a dog scheduled to be put down at a regional county animal shelter. The veterinarians in charge were

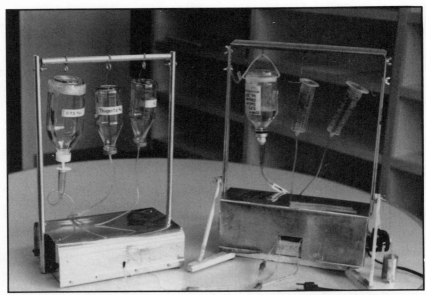

Figure 4. *Right*: The first Mercitron (used by Janet Adkins in June), after it was released by police. *Left*: A newer, as yet unused model.

willing to cooperate but suggested that I also get the permission of the head of the public health department. He in turn referred me to the local humane society, where I was told by the veterinarian there to put my request in writing so that it could be forwarded to the next policy board meeting four weeks hence.

I protested mildly that I merely wanted to use the device to substitute for routine hand injection of lethal agents. The obstinate reply was that the use of such a device would constitute an experiment and therefore would have to be approved by yet another special research ethics committee at its next meeting.

Disheartened by what I could easily guess to be expected of those committees' assessments, I made a last-ditch try with officials in a neighboring county—the same exasperating result occurred. Thoroughly frustrated, I exclaimed that it seemed as though I would have to use the device first to kill a doomed human being to prove that it is safe for killing a doomed animal!

On reflection, however, I came to the conclusion that rather than having been a setback, rejection of my request actually saved me from a serious breach of what I personally consider to be correct conduct in clinical research. That is, never to do on any live animal anything aimed solely or primarily for human benefit, and for the performance of which live human subjects are available under ethically unassailable circumstances.

That was the case when, in the early 1960s, I carried out cadaver blood transfusions only on human recipients, even for the first time. After all, the Russians had been doing it clinically for over forty years. I did not doubt their reports. In view of the extensive Russian experience with humans, there was no need for animal studies; yet, at the same time, a university-affiliated American research team squandered research funds to go to Moscow to observe the Russians at work, and returned home to experiment with cadaver blood transfusions on rabbits! Fortunately, I happened to be among unbiased and enthusiastic laboratorians, and employed at the only institution in the country (the Pontiac, Michigan, General Hospital) where such "controversial" research was permitted on humans.[110]

Two years later, in 1963, two collaborators helped me push ahead of the Russians by performing the first blood transfusions by syringe directly from cadavers to live human recipients—also without animal studies.[111] Because this innovation has immediate utility on battlefields, I applied for a federal grant to continue the research, even under combat conditions in Vietnam, if need be. My request was denied, and I resolved never again to waste time and effort in futile appeals for support from governmental agencies.

The biggest hurdle of all still faced me: access to the suffering patients who would want to use the device I had to offer. And they are many. Cruelly kept ignorant of my long-overdue option, patients are often compelled to improvise harsh means to end their wretched conditions. As proof one need only take a look at the awful tragedy on a national scale during just one week, as summarized in the 17 July 1989 issue of TIME magazine. Of a total of 464 cases of homicide in the United States by gunshot alone, 46 (10%) were self-inflicted to end the agony of some kind of terminal or crippling medical condition (excluding those of a purely psychiatric nature).

In line with known demographic trends, all but six of these suicides were men, ages twenty-four to eighty-seven (average age was sixty-five). The six women ranged in age from sixty-two to eighty-one (average age was seventy-two). The precipitating conditions included tumors and cancer, heart and lung diseases, diabetes, painful arthritis, stroke, cystic fibrosis, and Parkinson's disease. A few were listed simply as failing, poor, deterioriating or ill health; terminal disease; and avoidance of a nursing home or hospice.

The enormity of this sad state of affairs is magnified by the fact that all of these medical suicides were by gunshot only, and carried out only by those with the fortitude to tolerate and follow through with such a violent act. (That may be one reason, among others, why gun-related suicides of males far outnumber similar suicides for females.) Without much doubt there were many other suffering patients, men as well as women, who either resorted to other less violent means of death during that one week, or who involuntarily continued to suffer due to their own inability to use the means or to secure the necessary assistance.

One thing is sure: the autonomous decision to end physical suffering and the mental anguish that goes with it account for far more than ten percent of all homicides in the United States. Extrapolated to cover the full year, the published one week's toll would approximate two thousand patient suicides annually—by gunshot alone. Yet the medical profession doesn't care.

But I do, and I was more determined than ever to let patients know it. Classified ads in daily newspapers two years earlier were ineffective, let alone somewhat demeaning. So, I decided to once again challenge the medical press—surely another futile move. In late July 1989, I submitted to the editor of the Oakland County (Michigan) Medical Society *Bulletin* my proposed advertisement aimed at informing colleagues—as is customary among doctors—of the establishment of my new ethical practice of assisted suicide. It was rejected with this terse statement: "The physicians of the Oakland County Medical

Society are bound by oath to preserve life and do not endorse assisted suicide." This dubious refusal was certainly symptomatic of the medical community's fear in these matters.

Although still only theoretical, my unique practice interested the news department of a local television station. As a result, I and my device received valuable publicity during an evening newscast. Yet the lack of immediate response from the viewing audience was disconcerting.

Once again a direct personal appeal to individual oncologists seemed to be in order. It surprised me that a few of them were not aware that the panel in New York had declared the practice of assisted suicide for terminal patients to be ethical. But most were aware, and that made them more receptive to my inquiry, and made me less of a pariah in their eyes. For the first time, in October 1989, and at my own request, I was officially invited to address the weekly staff meeting of a local group of about sixty cancer specialists, many of whom were on a medical school faculty.

The reception was cordial but reserved and cool; the lingering fear and reticence were still evident. It was obvious that none of them yet had the temerity to let their dying patients partake of the new service. Nevertheless, the formal opportunity to air my views was one of those small successes I have come to appreciate.

Meanwhile, about ten days after the television publicity a young lady contacted me in behalf of her father, who was dying of lung cancer. They had seen the telecast and mulled the matter over for several days while "checking me out." Of course, their skepticism was understandable. Shortly thereafter, her father telephoned to make arrangements for a personal meeting to discuss details.

The forty-seven-year-old man was obviously very ill: thin, pale, emaciated, and in need of help to walk—even then his gait was slow and unsteady. His medical history was tragically brief. Normally a cheerful and active outdoorsman, in March 1989 he noted a slight but persistent pain in the right upper back, which eventually proved to be caused by inoperable cancer.

He wished to avoid death through semicoma induced by large doses of pain killers. I explained exactly what I could do for him and showed him pictures of the device to be used. Because chemotherapy was now out of the question, he definitely decided to die while still alert and mentally well-oriented. I consulted with his surgeon, who confirmed the patient's clinical story. Although the surgeon would not condone or take part in my planned procedure, he admitted that it probably was the best course of action.

At the patient's request, I met with him and his family at his home the next evening. Having been bedridden since our first meeting ten days earlier, he was now noticeably more lethargic as a result of heavy medication. He soon dozed off as I conversed with his mother, former wife, son, and daughter. About a half an hour later I was quite relieved to see him awake, alert, and willing to sign an informed consent to verify his determination to proceed as planned. The other family members signed a statement attesting to the patient's mental competency.

Under extraordinary circumstances like these I feel it is only decent and fair to explain my ultimate aim. I emphasized that it is not simply to help suffering or doomed persons kill themselves—that is merely the first step, an early distasteful professional obligation (now called medicide) that nobody in his or her right mind could savor. I explained that what I find most satisfying is the prospect of making possible the performance of invaluable experiments or other beneficial medical acts under conditions that this first unpleasant step can help establish—in a word, obitiatry, as defined earlier.

Rather than finding my elaboration to be unacceptably macabre, everyone in the room extolled my aim without reservation. And something else happened to confirm what I suspected would be a favorable by-product of the new option. It seems that the mere knowledge of the availability, or just the anticipation of making use, of doctor-assisted suicide has a strangely salubrious effect on patients, as though adding zest to what little life remains. When I got up to leave, the man was clearly more alert and at ease despite his pain and languor—and in an astoundingly jovial frame of mind, he cracked jokes as I exited toward my car.

At this session, as when I first met the patient, I repeatedly warned that I could be of service only if he was conscious and coherent. It was obvious that very little time remained. Nevertheless he wished to postpone the procedure for two weeks in order to see his son off on a vacation. The son reinforced my doubts about the wisdom of his father's decision, saying that he most likely would not be taking the trip because of the latter's imminent death. Our doubts were borne out two days later when the patient unexpectedly slipped into babbling incoherence. That eliminated him as the first candidate for my services.

With this "near miss" I had taken the first tiny step in the transformation of an undoubtedly correct abstract concept into an equally correct concrete reality. But I knew that it would take a "bulls-eye" to establish the new specialty, which meant that I had to find a more effective way to make known the availability of this new service.

All local newspapers refused to take a paid display ad. Luckily, a feature writer at the *Oakland Press* in Pontiac, Michigan, found my campaign to be interesting and asked me in for a personal interview in preparation for a feature article. I brought along the Mercitron, and a picture of me and the device appeared with the article in October 1989.

A *Detroit News* reporter, who saw the article, immediately requested a similar interview and photograph. When this second article was published and sent over the wire services, I was deluged for days with numerous requests to take part in radio and television call-in talk shows in many states. The audience response was extremely favorable, and I received many pleas for help from suffering patients, locally and in other states. Unfortunately, most of those states have laws that prohibit assisting a suicide under penalty of imprisonment.

The widespread publicity led to a telephone call from a forty-five-year-old woman near Detroit, crippled by severe multiple sclerosis (MS). Speaking in a subdued, dejected voice, she expressed a firm desire to end her life of deepening misery over the previous fifteen years. Confined to a wheelchair with complete paralysis of both legs and one arm and near complete paralysis of the other arm, she needed constant assistance in performing even the simplest routine tasks of daily living.

I requested the name of her neurologist in order to notify him immediately of her extraordinary request. The news shocked him. (It is astonishing how little some doctors know—or seem to care— about what their patients really think or feel.) After recovering from the initial jolt, the neurologist agreed to meet with me, his patient, and her closest relative (a twenty-one-year-old daughter) in his office four days later.

Despite the gloomy topic and circumstances, the consultation went surprising well—quite low-key and without manifest emotionalism. Seated in her motorized wheelchair, the patient slowly and softly reiterated her desire to die. She admitted having mulled the idea over for a long time, but decided to proceed only when her daughter's impending graduation from college seemed to assure the latter's prospects for an independent livelihood.

The neurologist verified the patient's clinical condition in detail. Although he could not condone her planned action, he did concede that patients have a right to come to such a decision, and that there is a need for this kind of medical intervention. His honest, commonsense attitude was especially welcome and gratifying.

Even more gratifying was the gradual, almost imperceptible change in his patient's demeanor during our forty-five minute meeting. Slowly her dour countenance turned serene. To help put her mind at ease I repeatedly assured her that I would always be ready to help end her misery, no matter what anyone else says or thinks—that the decision was hers alone. Because her condition was not imminently lethal and there was no need for hasty action, I seconded the neurologist's suggestion that she try another, somewhat modified therapy regimen, though the prospect did not appeal to her. Despite obvious skepticism she agreed to give it a try. Also at my suggestion, the neurologist referred her for psychiatric evaluation with regard to possible depression. I was amazed that he had neglected to take that logical step (not to mention that it was a fundamental professional obligation).

The patient's acquiescence seemed to be a direct consequence of unexpected equanimity. Her facial expression showed less anxiety as the discussion wore on, and her overall composure less lassitude.

There was no doubt that the assurance of having been offered the option of competent and professionally assisted suicide eased her panic-stricken mind, thereby diverting much of her otherwise wasted mental energy into constructive channels. This was manifested by a most favorable sign: near the end of our discussion, and for the first time, a faint smile crossed her face as she promised to undergo the special course of treatment. I was convinced that she was not in the grip of morbid depression.

Subsequent experience with other suffering patients has reinforced my conviction that such a favorable impact of medicide might be widespread. I have received numerous supportive letters and telephone calls from many adults, both ill and healthy, of all ages, and from many states. In several instances the agonized individuals told me that they decided to go on with more treatment when assured of the availability of the Mercitron as a last resort. Two elderly, physically healthy women expressed great mental relief in having the same assurance. One of them tearfully vouched that the mere existence of my device had relieved her of constant worry over future disability, and that now she could enjoy peace of mind for the first time in many years.

From these reactions I have concluded that if offered as a legitimate medical service everywhere, medicide would soon reduce substantially the increasing rate of suicide for all age groups, especially the elderly. It has been proven that most suicides result from panic, perhaps due to the terror of seeing no way out of a dilemma, and compounded by the bewildering pangs of trying to decide how and where one is to kill oneself. Medicide can eliminate, or at least ameliorate, the lethal panic by reinforcing the "safety valve" mentioned by Williams and alluded to in chapter 13. Thus assured of the opportunity for humane, dignified, and easily accessible suicide, a *naturally tranquilized* mind can then concentrate on more rational and positive behavior, which would preclude such drastic action. For the first time in history medicide would offer the objective means of distinguishing rational from irrational suicide. After all, with that option at hand, would anyone *in his or her right mind* "choose" (that is, be driven by panic) instead to commit suicide by other ordinary, messy, and usually violent means?

In most cases of those who requested information or pleaded for assisted suicide—and the letters and calls came from all parts of the country (and a few foreign countries)—I could only commiserate or lend verbal support, because medicide was a felony or a capital crime in the political jurisdictions concerned. Many of those who called and wrote to me seethed with bitterness and contempt toward society and its medical profession, blaming physicians for the deplorable state of affairs. I wonder if doctors realize just how deep the public resentment runs. I also wonder if they would care much even if they were aware of it. The insouciance of organized medicine seems to belie an attitude of "benevolence," which at its root is arbitrary and strictly self-serving.

The crippled MS patient telephoned again in December 1989 to inform me that the latest course of therapy failed to arrest her deterioration. With increasing pain in the hips and back due to a twisted spine, she pleaded for assistance in ending her life. I notified her neurologist at once, and he concurred that I should arrange for a second personal interview with her as soon as possible.

In the meantime the producers of a nationally syndicated television news and documentary program learned of my activities and requested permission to videotape separate interviews with me to display my device, and later the same day with the MS patient at her apartment. The following day the program's host telephoned to tell me that during his interview the patient expressed an unequivocal wish to die and end her suffering.

My second meeting with her took place at her apartment in late December 1989. My sister was also present and helped sustain a wide-ranging discussion. We encouraged the patient to overcome her reluctance to share her plans and feelings openly with a wider circle of friends and relatives, and to explore alternatives that might make life more bearable before resorting to the finality of suicide. Her extreme debility was obvious as we watched her fumble through the simple task of handling the telephone to answer a call that had interrupted our discussion. Eventually we came to the main reason for my visit.

I had to make the patient understand why she was not a suitable candidate for the first use of the Mercitron. Even though she was terribly agonized by an intolerable "quality of life," her condition was not imminently terminal. In order to minimize the passionate (if irrational) storm of criticism certain to be evoked by such a procedure, I realized that ideally it should be in connection with a suffering and indisputably terminal patient—for example, someone dying of incurable and widespread cancer. I explained how that should blunt condemnation of my assisting her as the second case. Despite disappointment at the incessant postponements, she understood and held me to a promise to help her immediately after the initial event.

Several weeks later she agreed to appear before television and newspaper reporters at her home to announce her readiness to use the Mercitron. However, one of her relatives suddenly appeared, blocked access to her apartment, and later that day secretly whisked her off to a large medical center. Shortly thereafter I received word that she wanted me to contact her at the hospital, but she had no access to a telephone. I learned from her daughter that after having been released from the hospital earlier, the patient failed in a suicide attempt at home and was rehospitalized incommunicado. I never heard from her again.

The telecast in January 1990 of our previously videotaped interviews elicited another spate of supportive responses from around the country. Among them was a local call from another forty-one-year-old woman afflicted with severe MS. I arranged to meet the woman, her parents, and her neurologist at the physician's office located in a large medical center in Detroit. Confined to a wheelchair and with very limited use of one arm only, the pretty but frail and emaciated little female figure was a pitiable sight—a far cry from the robust, talented dancer and skater of earlier years. It was obvious that her neurologist disagreed emphatically with her wishes. Somewhat reluctantly he discussed her clinical history and condition with me and admitted that he knew of nothing more that he could do to arrest her deterioration, which had been progressive and constant for ten years. He left the room as quickly as possible when I began talking with the parents. They, too, disapproved of her wish to end her life, but despite ambivalence and sadness they appreciated their daughter's deep anguish and acknowledged the primacy of her self-determination.

It is almost incredible that in this instance, as was the case with the first MS patient, her neurologist decided to refer her for psychiatric consultation for the first time only after I broached the subject during our clinical discussion.

The patient's unwavering determination to end her suffering was certified beyond doubt when she subsequently marshaled the courage to announce it to the world on local and national telecasts here and in Canada. She did so more for the sake of the concept and to help others in similar circumstances than to draw attention to her own plight. And as her condition continued to worsen to the point of almost total helplessness, she knew that she would not qualify as the first candidate for the Mercitron.

15

The Birth of Medicide

Amid the flurry of telephone calls in the fall of 1989 was one from a man in Portland, Oregon, who learned of my campaign from an item in *Newsweek* (November 13, 1989). Ron Adkins's rich, baritone, matter-of-fact voice was tinged with a bit of expectant anxiety as he calmly explained the tragic situation of his beloved wife. Janet Adkins was a remarkable, accomplished, active woman—wife, mother, grandmother, revered friend, teacher, musician, mountain climber, and outdoorsperson—who, for some time, had noticed (as did her husband) subtle and gradually progressive impairment of her memory. The shock of hearing the diagnosis of Alzheimer's disease four months earlier was magnified by the abrupt and somewhat callous way her doctor announced it. The intelligent woman knew what the diagnosis portended, and at that instant decided she would not live to experience the horror of such a death.

Knowing that Janet was a courageous fighter, Ron and their three sons pleaded with her to reconsider and at least give a promising new therapy regimen a try. Ron explained to me that Janet was eligible to take part in an experimental trial using the newly developed drug Tacrine® or THA* at the University of Washington in Seattle. I concurred that Janet should enroll in the program because any candidate for the Mercitron must have exhausted every potentially beneficial medical intervention, no matter how remotely promising.

I heard nothing more from the Adkinses until April 1990. Ron called again, after Janet and he saw me and my device on a nationally televised talk show. Janet had entered the experimental program in January, but it had been stopped early because the new drug was ineffective. In fact, her condition got worse; and she was more determined than ever to end her life. Even though from a physical standpoint Janet was not imminently terminal, there seemed little doubt that mentally she was—and, after all, it is one's mental status that determines the essence of one's existence. I asked Ron to forward to me copies of Janet's clinical records, and they corroborated what Ron had said.

I then telephoned Janet's doctor in Seattle. He opposed her planned action and the concept of assisted suicide in general. It was his firm opinion that Janet would remain mentally competent for at least a year (but from Ron's narrative I concluded that her doctor's opinion was wrong and that time was of the essence). Because Janet's condition was deteriorating and there was nothing else that might help arrest it, I decided to accept her as the first candidate—a qualified, justifiable candidate if not "ideal"—and well aware of the vulnerability to criticism of picayune and overly emotional critics.

A major obstacle was finding a place to do it. Because I consider medicide to be necessary, ethical, and legal, there should be nothing furtive about it. Another reason to pursue the practice above-board is to avert the harrassment or vindictiveness of litigation. Consequently, when searching for a suitable site I always explained that I planned to assist a suffering patient to commit suicide. That posed no problem

---

*1, 2, 3, 4—Tetrahydro—9—acridinamine

for helping a Michigan resident in his or her own residence. But it was a different matter for an out-of-state guest who must rent temporary quarters.

And I soon found out how difficult a matter it could be. My own apartment could not be used because of lease constraints, and the same was true of my sister's apartment. I inquired at countless motels, funeral homes, churches of various denominations, rental office buildings, clinics, doctors' offices for lease, and even considered the futile hope of renting an emergency life-support ambulance. Many owners, proprietors, and landlords were quite sympathetic but fearful and envisioned the negative public reaction that could seriously damage and even destroy their business enterprises. In short, they deemed it bad for public relations. More dismaying yet was the refusal of people who are known supporters and active campaigners for euthanasia to allow Janet and me the use of their homes.

Finally, a friend agreed to avail us of his modest home in Detroit; I immediately contacted Ron to finalize plans. My initial proposal was to carry out the procedure at the end of May 1990, but Ron and Janet preferred to avoid the surge of travel associated with the Memorial Day weekend. The date was postponed to Monday, June 4th.

In the meantime, my friend was warned by a doctor, in whom he confided, not to make his home available for such a purpose. Soon thereafter the offer was quickly withdrawn. With the date set and airline tickets having been purchased by Janet, Ron, and a close friend of Janet's, I had to scamper to find another site. The device required an electrical outlet, which limited the possibilities.

I had made a Herculean effort to provide a desirable, clinical setting. Literally and sadly, there was "no room at the inn." Now, having been refused everywhere I applied, the *only alternative* remaining was my 1968 camper (see figure 5) and a suitable campground.

As expected, the owners of a commercial site refused permission, even though they were sympathetic to the proposed scheme. They then suggested the solution by recommending that I rent space at a public camping site not too far away. The setting was pleasant and idyllic.

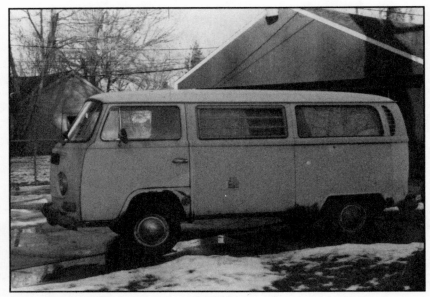

Figure 5. My 1968 camper—January 1991.

As with many other aspects of this extraordinary event, I was aware of the harsh criticism that would be leveled at the use of a "rusty old van." In the first place, the twenty-two-year-old body may have been rusting on the outside, but its interior was very clean, orderly, and comfortable. I have slept in it often and not felt degraded. But carping critics missed the point: the essence and significance of the event are far more important than the splendor of the site where it takes place. If critics are thus deluded into denouncing the exit from existence under these circumstances, then why not the same delusional denunciation of entrance into existence when a baby is, of necessity, born in an old taxicab? On the contrary, the latter identical scenario seems to arouse only feelings of sentimental reverence and quaint joy.

But the dishonesty doesn't stop there. I have been repeatedly criticized for having assisted a patient after a short personal acquaintance of two days. Overlooked or ignored is my open avowal to be the first practitioner in this country of a new and as yet officially unrecognized specialty. Because of shameful stonewalling by her own doctors, Janet was forced to refer herself to me. And acting as a unique specialist, of necessity self-proclaimed, solitary, and independent, I was obligated to scrutinize Janet's clinical records and to consult with her personal doctor. The latter's uncooperative attitude (tacitly excused by otherwise harsh critics) impaired but did not thwart fulfillment of my duties to a suffering patient and to my profession.

It is absurd even to imply, let alone to protest outright, that a medical specialist's competence and ethical behavior are contingent upon some sort of time interval, imposed arbitrarily or by fiat. When a doctor refers a patient for surgery, in many cases the surgical specialist performs his *ultimate* duty after personal acquaintance with the patient from a mere hour or two of prior consultation (in contrast to my having spent at least twelve hours in personal contact with Janet). In a few instances the surgeon operates on a patient seen for the first time on the operating table—and anesthetized to unconsciousness.

Moreover, in sharp contrast to the timorous, secretive, and even deceitful intention and actions of other medical euthanasists on whom our so-called bioethicists now shower praise, I acted openly, ethically, legally, with complete and uncompromising honesty, and—even more important—I remained in personal attendance during the second most meaningful medical event in a patient's earthly existence. Were he alive today, it's not hard to guess what Hippocrates would say about all this.

My two sisters, Margo and Flora, and I met with Ron, Janet, and Janet's close friend Carroll Rehmke in their motel room on Saturday afternoon, 2 June 1990 (see figure 6). After getting acquainted through a few minutes of conversation, the purpose of the trip was thoroughly discussed. I had already prepared authorization forms signifying Janet's intent, determination, and freedom of choice, which she readily agreed to sign. Here again, while she was resolute in her decision, and absolutely mentally competent, her impaired memory was apparent when she needed her husband's assistance in forming the cursive letter "A." She could print the letter but not write it, and the consent forms required that her signature be written. So her

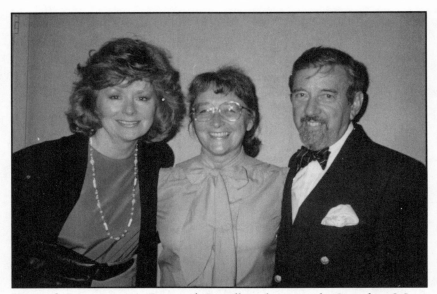

Figure 6. Janet (center), Ron and Carroll at their motel—Saturday, 2 June 1990

husband showed her on another piece of paper how to form the cursive "A," and Janet complied. At this time, Ron and Carroll also signed a statement attesting to Janet's mental competence. Following this signing session, I had Flora videotape my interview with Janet and Ron. The forty-five-minute taping reinforced my own conviction that Janet was mentally competent but that her memory had failed badly. However, the degree of memory failure led me to surmise that within four to six months she would be too incompetent to qualify as a candidate. It should be pointed out that in medical terms loss of memory does not automatically signify mental incompetence. Any rational critic would concede that a mentally sound individual can be afflicted with even total amnesia.

Around 5:30 P.M. that same day all six of us had dinner at a well-known local restaurant. Seated around the same table for many hours, our conversation covered many subjects, including the telling of jokes. Without appearing too obvious, I constantly observed Janet's behavior and assessed her moods as well as the content and quality of her thoughts. There was absolutely no doubt that her mentality was intact and that she was not the least depressed over her impending death. On the contrary, the only detectable anxiety or disquieting demeanor was among the rest of us to a greater or lesser degree. Even in response to jokes, Janet's appropriately timed and modulated laughter indicated clear and coherent comprehension. The only uneasiness or distress she exhibited was due to her embarrassment at being unable to recall aspects of the topic under discussion at the time. And that is to be expected of intelligent, sensitive, and diligent individuals.

We left the restaurant at 12:30 A.M. Sunday. Janet and Ron enjoyed their last full day by themselves.

At 8:30 A.M. the next day, Monday, 4 June 1990, I drove into a rented space at Groveland Park in north Oakland County, Michigan. At the same time, my sisters drove to the motel to fetch Janet, who had composed (and submitted to my sister) a brief and clear note reiterating her genuine desire to end her life and exonerating all others in this desire and the actual event (see figure 7). For the last time, Janet took tearful leave of her grieving husband and Carroll, both of whom were inconsolable. It was Janet's wish that they not accompany her to the park.

The day began cold, damp, and overcast. I took a lot of time in setting up the Mercitron and giving it a few test runs. In turning to get a pair of pliers in the cramped space within the van, I accidentally knocked over the container of thiopental solution, losing a little over half of it. I was fairly sure that the remainder was enough to induce and maintain adequate unconsciousness, but I chose not to take the risk. I drove the forty-five miles home and got some more.

In the meantime, at about 9:30 A.M. my sisters and Janet had arrived at the park. They were dismayed to learn of the accidental spill and opted to accompany me on the extra round trip, which required two and one-half hours. We reentered the park at approximately noontime. Janet remained in the car with Margo while Flora helped me with minor tasks in the van as I very carefully prepared and tested the Mercitron. Everything was ready by about 2:00 P.M., and Janet was summoned.

I have decided for the following reason to take my own life. This is a decision taken in a normal state of mind and is fully considered

I have alzheimers disease and do not want to let it progress any further. I dont choose to put my family or myself through the agony of this Terrible disease.

Janet E. Adkins

June 4ᵗʰ 1990

WITNESS: Carroll Rehmke   June 4ᵗʰ 1990
Ronald Adkins   June 4ᵗʰ 1990

Figure 7. Janet Adkins's final note, written on the morning of her death.

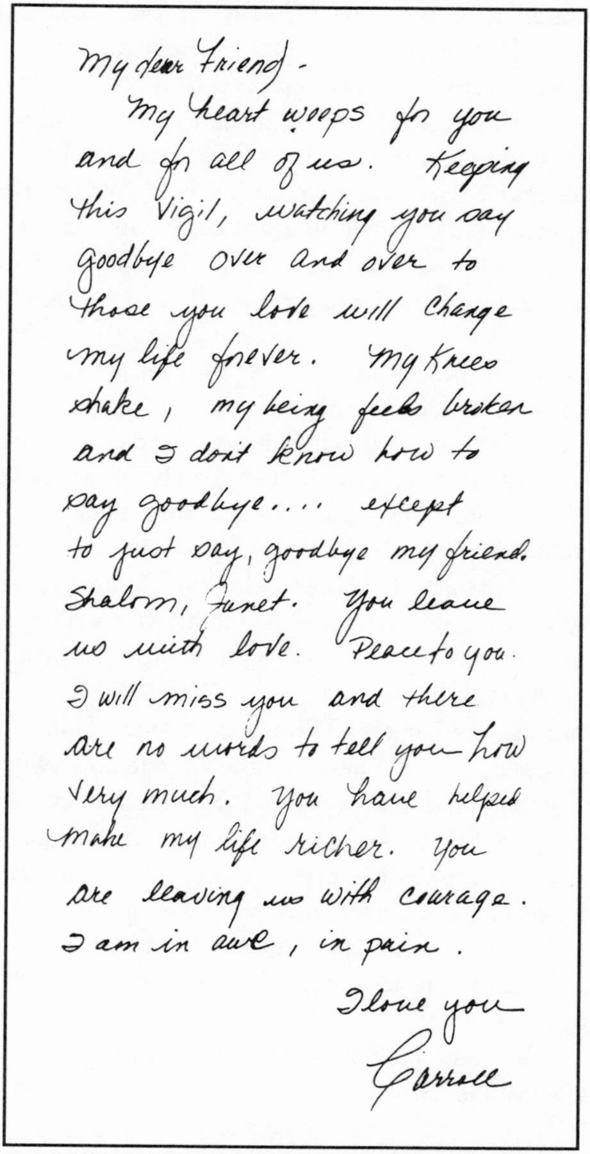

My dear Friend -

My heart weeps for you and for all of us. Keeping this Vigil, watching you say goodbye over and over to those you love will change my life forever. My Knees shake, my being feels broken and I don't know how to say goodbye.... except to just say, goodbye my friend. Shalom, Janet. You leave us with love. Peace to you. I will miss you and there are no words to tell you how very much. You have helped make my life richer. You are leaving us with courage. I am in awe, in pain.

I love you

Carroll

Figure 8. Carroll's note written on 4 June 1990 and read by my sister to Janet in the camper a few minutes before Janet pressed the switch.

She entered the van alone through the open sliding side door and lay fully clothed on the built-in bed covered with freshly laundered sheets. Her head rested comfortably on a clean pillow. The windows were covered with new draperies. With Janet's permission I cut small holes in her nylon stockings at the ankles, attached ECG electrodes to her ankles and wrists, and covered her body with a light blanket. Our conversation was minimal. In accordance with Janet's wish, Flora read to her a brief note from her friend Carroll (see figure 8), followed by a reading of the Lord's prayer. I then repeated my earlier instructions to Janet about how the device was to be activated, and asked her to go through the motions. In contrast to my sister and me, Janet was calm and outwardly relaxed.

I used a syringe with attached needle to pierce a vein near the frontal elbow area of her left arm. Unfortunately, her veins were delicate and fragile; even slight movement of the restrained arm caused the needle to penetrate through the wall of the vein resulting in leakage. Two more attempts also failed, as did a fourth attempt on the right side. Finally an adequte puncture was obtained on the right arm. (It was reassuring to me to learn later that doctors in Seattle had had similar difficulty with her veins.)

The moment had come. With a nod from Janet I turned on the ECG and said, "Now." Janet hit the Mercitron's switch with the outer edge of her palm. In about ten seconds her eyelids began to flicker and droop. She looked up at me and said, "Thank you, thank you." I replied at once as her eyelids closed, "Have a nice trip." She was unconscious and perfectly still except for two widely spaced and mild coughs several minutes later. Agonal complexes in the ECG tracing indicated death due to complete cessation of blood circulation in six minutes.

It was 2:30 P.M. Suddenly—for the first time that cold, dank day—warm sunshine bathed the park.

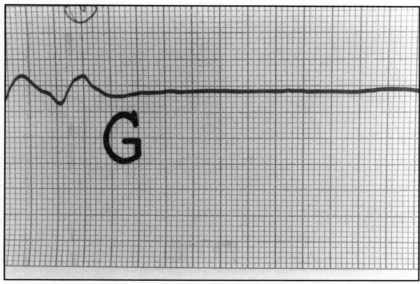

Figure 9. ECG lead AVF (electrode on right ankle): agonal complexes, with arrest, circulation ended.

16

Prognosis: Medicide
Positive or Negative?

Flora and I had witnessed an epochal event that will refocus the moral dimensions of purposeful termination of human life, raising it from pointless disputation over merely nihilistic "mercy killing" or judicial execution to a higher plane of respectability due the promise of obitiatry. The inferences to be drawn from this first actual experience with honorable medicide are enormous and their significance incalculable.

First of all, no longer is there a need—or even an excuse—for anyone to be the direct mediator of the death of another who is alert, rational, and who for some compelling reason chooses to, or must, die. Performance of that repulsive task should now be relegated exclusively to a device like the Mercitron, which the doomed subject must activate. What is most important is that the participation of doctors or other health professionals now becomes strictly

233

optional, either to insert a needle into the subject's vein to start the harmless saline infusion, or to monitor an ECG tracing to verify and document the occurrence of death. A doctor no longer need perform the injection.

Such indirect and innocuous (and to some extent even beneficial) medical conduct concentrates any question of morality only, and squarely, on the patient. Morality thus so absolutely subjectivized is hopelessly immune to justifiable extraneous (or objective) assessment. In other words, it is wrong for any and all members of society to even try to judge the morality of an individual's action, deemed by that society to be immoral, when the individual concerned disagrees and performs the action in such a manner as not to infringe the autonomy of others or society's official rules of culpability.

Euthanasia for conscious, mentally competent patients—in a word, medicide—has now been eliminated as an ethical problem for the medical profession everywhere except in the Netherlands. That refreshingly vibrant medical community will soon, and quite unexpectedly and undeservedly, find itself in a moral quandary demanding an about-face.

Heretofore the majority of Dutch doctors endorsed as ethical their involvement with active euthanasia currently condemned by conventional medical ethics. But the Mercitron now undeniably makes such conduct by doctors (or anyone else) vulnerable to moral censure. To avoid it, all euthanasists in the Netherlands eventually, and the sooner the better, will have to stop practicing active euthanasia, and instead merely help patients accomplish it themselves with the aid of the Mercitron.

The device's impact on morality extends to execution chambers as well. The same moral vulnerability applies directly to the one unknown executioner who voluntarily (albeit unwittingly) injects a lethal drug mixture into a condemned criminal's vein; and indirectly to the society that orders the injection. Only by using the Mercitron to carry out those lethal injections can the stigma of moral vulnerability be erased—and, as you will see, the execution made even more humane.

The current procedure of judicial lethal injection need hardly be altered. Someone must perform a venipuncture on the condemned to start the I.V. saline drip. The rest would be up to the Mercitron. Onset of the flow of lethal solutions would be controlled by a small switch, perhaps in an adjacent room, to be activated by an unseen executioner.

As now practiced, lethal injection requires several individuals to use multiple syringes of fluid, only one of which actually contains the lethal mixture. That is designed to minimize feelings of guilt on the part of the executioners in the same way that the use of one blank cartridge in a firing squad is supposed to diffuse moral guilt.

The Mercitron can diffuse it even more by eliminating entirely the need for anyone to inject anything. Out of view of the execution scene, five "executioners" will simply press five identical buttons making the same "click," but only one of which starts the lethal flow. That kind of indirect, passive involvement ameliorates moral responsibility a bit further. And with one additional, relatively minor modification of the procedure, the Mercitron would not only reduce moral vulnerability on the part of executioners to near zero, but also would make the entire procedure more humane.

You may be wondering how that can be, how such a simple device can promise so much. Consider this suggestion: grant the condemned the privilege of choosing to activate the Mercitron themselves. That extra nuance of respect, deserved or not, for the personal autonomy of the condemned is what would enhance the humaneness of the act and the moral integrity of the society responsible for it.

There is little doubt in my mind that some, perhaps most, condemned individuals would welcome that option, at least for the satisfaction of having a tiny measure of control over the immediate circumstances and processes of their own deaths. For proof I decided to ask five of the men on death row with whom I have been corresponding what they thought of the suggestion. As of this writing (March 1991) four of the five have responded.

The first opinion came from Joseph Roger O'Dell, III, in Virginia: "The answer is YES I would. I think that a condemned man can be analogized with a person that is terminally ill . . . and I think that if they are going to die, then they should have the option as to the way they will die. My personal opinion is that your invention is very humane. . . . You certainly have my endorsement."

From Mitchell Terry Mincey in Georgia came these comments: "I'm in favor of your idea/device because I think there are many people who would like to use it. Given a chance I would ask for it at my execution just so I could deprive some gung-ho guard of the chance. And since I want to donate my organs, I think it would help further that desire by removing the responsibility from those who object to killing me for the use of organs. . . . I fully support this idea, too."

Richard Norman Rojem, Jr., in Oklahoma, had reservations. He wrote: "Personally, no, I would not like the option. I may go to my death like a man, but I don't think I could help the State carry out the execution by relieving them of the burden. That is not to say that some wouldn't do it themselves, but when you consider the suicide rate on the row, nationwide, chances are not too many would be agreeable."

Jonathan Nobles, now on death row in Texas, was equally reluctant. "I don't know what to say about your device. I guess to each his own, but for me I would not consider it an option."

The fact that two of the four inmates gave my suggestion outright endorsement is irrefutable proof that it is on target and should receive serious consideration if not immediate implementation by penal authorities. Even Rojem conceded that others might welcome the privilege of choice even though he personally does not endorse it, and he is willing to see it offered to them in spite of his own feelings.

The option would be neither unique nor innovative. Back in the fourth century B.C. a genuinely respectful Greek society honored one of its most illustrious condemned "criminals" by sparing Socrates the ignominy of an executioner's sword. Instead he was granted the privilege of choosing to kill himself with relative dignity by calmly drinking poison in the company of friends and at a time of his choosing.

With the Mercitron has arisen the obligation of our society to show whether or not it wants to rise to a similar level of enlightenment in the implementation of the death penalty. From my experience I would guess that for the foreseeable future our society would prefer to remain content at its current comfortable level somewhat down the scale.

But that does not bar me from calling society's bluff. If the condemned who wish to kill themselves at an officially set time are denied by society the privilege of activating the extant means (such as the Mercitron) for a humane and rapid death, if they are forced to have death *inflicted*, then society's motives may well harbor more intent than simply making sure that a capital transgressor's life is ended. The extra concern over how it is done and who is to do it could justify suspicion that society deceitfully keeps open the possibility of imbuing even the most humane method with a gratifying touch of revenge. Could that not also imply a touch of sadism?

In the final analysis, the thwarting of a condemned individual's last chance to exercise the personal autonomy of free choice concerning the second most profound moment in life can denote nothing other than a society bent on perpetuating the psychic cruelty associated with capital punishment (as we discussed in chapter 4)—a society addicted to the gratification of a hopelessly ineffaceable lust for revenge.

Whether for patients or the condemned, it all boils down to negative euthanasia. As I have already mentioned, even the Mercitron is not the complete answer. But it provides the all-important first small step toward the ultimate goal of *positive medicide*, which obitiatry alone can achieve. Only then will society have achieved real progress toward enlightenment.

17

Completing the Medical Spectrum

Traditionally the mission of a healer has been to ease pain and suffering as well as to preserve and restore health and, as corollaries, to facilitate birth and to postpone death. The latter two cardinal events mark off what I call the "visible spectrum" of medicine, the components of which fluctuated very little if at all from antiquity to the recent past.

In view of the early rudimentary knowledge of human biology with its plethora of herbs and drugs having little or no efficacy, of fanciful dietary regimens, of a few crude surgical procedures, and the psychological impact of doctors' priestly aura, it is understandable why the amplitude and intensity of that "visible spectrum" remained relatively invariable and small for many centuries. Throughout the world, human beings of all ages were constantly at the mercy of crippling and lethal diseases occurring sporadically or as devastating plagues, and against which a weak medical arsenal had very little to offer. In such bleak circumstances it is no small wonder that a desperate humanity would rank the maintenance and prolongation of life to be medicine's primary mission.

Other less mundane but equally important factors were involved in the establishment of that priority in the Western world. Perhaps the most powerful was the inflexible and harshly punitive Judeo-Christian dogma that espoused the absolute and inviolable "sanctity" of human life. Reinforcing that was the medieval necessity for powerful emperors and feudal lords to keep their personal combat forces adequately manned. Among the inevitable consequences of all this were the taboos against abortion, suicide, and euthanasia. Vestiges of those taboos have endured to our "enlightened" time.

The ironclad morality of such arbitrary rule ethics began to crack under the pressure of scientific, demographic, economic, and social changes. The rate of increase of population and of living standards became geometric as a result of advances in medical capabilities, in public health, and in the industrial transformation of agrarian cultures. These in turn secularized society and vitiated theistic absolutism. The ensuing pressures led to official breach of two of the taboos mentioned above. Within the last century the common law crime of suicide has been annulled; the act is no longer illegal. Abortion and birth control, too, have been legitimized, albeit intermittently and with limitations. No matter what legal or religious injunctions are imposed in the foreseeable future, these two taboos will never again withstand the evolving pressures of contrary demand. (The Prohibition fiasco should be lesson enough.)

The breaking of the stranglehold on practices of abortion and birth control not only enhanced one extreme of medicine's "visible spectrum" but also helped expand it into the previously unimagined and even unthinkable "ultrabirth" realm. An overdue lenity paved the way for the application of increasingly sophisticated techniques of modern science and technology in the evolution of a new specialty called fetology, and in expanding the frontiers of embryology. It is in this currently "invisible ultrabirth" part of the biological spectrum (analogous to the invisible ultraviolet component of the physical electromagnetic spectrum) that the promise of so-called genetic engineering will be realized. From the ashes of a shattered taboo will have arisen the best possible means to search for the cure or prevention of countless genetic and hereditary diseases—and even perhaps to preprogram every human conceptus for a long life of guaranteed biological integrity.

The time has come to smash the last irrational and most fearsome taboo of planned death and thereby to open the floodgates of equally momentous benefit for humankind. In the first place, and as emphasized repeatedly throughout this book, the positive euthanasia of obitiatry would expand enormously the amplitude and intensity of the ordinary "visible spectrum." It would do this by allowing doctors for the first time to carry out on living human beings otherwise impossible trials of new and untested drugs, devices, or operations. That would accelerate medical progress by eliminating the need for experiments on animals or on ill patients who volunteer to be test subjects. But the biggest impact of obitiatry will probably be its extension of the abstract spectrum of medicine into the opposite "invisible infradeath" realm, where the real potential for serious investigation of the phenomenon of death is to be found.

There will always be a demand for that sort of investigation as long as humans exist. This cannot be said with equal certainty in connection with the "visible spectrum" of conventional medical practice. Unforeseen sociopolitical and economic upheavals coupled with burgeoning populations may so strain resources as to limit or even reduce the necessity or demand for more sophisticated and very expensive medical care. That possibility is presaged by the current debate over the inevitable rationing of costly medical resources. But compared to the costs of setting up and maintaining ordinary healthcare facilities, those with regard to obitoria would be far less.

In the first place, because of their more limited and highly specialized purposes, relatively fewer obitoria with smaller staffs would be needed in any community setting. Ordinary medical costs now are spiraling out of control because of the innumerable and expensive services offered and the large numbers of people who partake of them. Neither of these factors would apply to an obitorium. But more than thrift alone enhances the prospects of longevity for obitiatry. Whether healthy, sick, or moribund, human beings will always ponder the mystery of death; and in itself that is enough to validate and maintain the existence of obitoria and the practice of positive medicide even when and if the demand for or availability of traditional medical care levels off, declines, or disappears altogether.

From a scientific standpoint death is an absolutely unfathomable mystery. But so, too, are birth and life (or existence itself). Nobody has even a hint of true knowledge about where we came from, where we now are, and where we will be when we die. Heretofore all research on death has consisted solely of objective descriptions of gross and microscopic morphological changes and chemical analyses associated with the biological deterioration of the physical body, and of the subjective, emotional, or psychological impact of impending demise. Neither approach yields any really objective knowledge about the subjective state or process called death.

That is also true of so-called near-death phenomena, which are nothing other than hallucinations caused by the irritative effect of cerebral anoxia (lack of oxygen to the brain) and obviously reversible.

It may be (and most likely is) true that the essence of birth, life, and death ultimately is far beyond the reach of science. After all, we humans have limited intellectual or reasoning powers wholly dependent on a flimsy perceptive mechanism composed of five extremely variable and certainly fallible senses, and a sixth very moot sense called intuition.

What does that mean in a universe of infinitude? Could there be many more senses, perhaps an infinite number of them, all qualitatively different, which humans don't have and can't even imagine, and which might characterize totally alien and inconceivable forms of existence in "spaces" and "times" perfectly congruous with ours and absolutely undetectable to one another? For example, it is by sight alone that we humans know of the existence of intact organisms called amebas (and that knowledge was only recently acquired). Does the ameba know of our existence as an intact organism? If so, how, and by what sense(s)? And for what strange and unimaginable "forms of existence" are *we* the "amebas"?

If we are ever to penetrate the mystery of death—even superficially—it will have to be through obitiatry. Research using cultured cells and tissues and live animals may yield objective biological data, and eventually perhaps even some clues about the essence of mere vitality or existence. But knowledge about the essence of human death will of necessity require insight into the nature of the unique awareness or consciousness that characterizes cognitive human *life*. That is possible only through obitiatric research on living human bodies, and most likely by concentrating on the central nervous system. Of course, the prerequisite of general anesthesia is an unavoidable drawback, but not a nullifying one. Just as the discovery of rapid eye movement (REM) during sleep proved to be a means for objectively detecting the otherwise unknowable occurrence and quality of subjective dreaming in an unconscious subject, so, too, may obitiatric research on anesthetized subjects yield comparable objective means to pinpoint the exact onset of extinction of an unknown cognitive mechanism that energizes life.

The "spectrum" of medicine may never be completed. Every scientific advance can be of no real consequence in the vastness of infinity. It seems that every generation of scientists sometimes comes to the foolish conclusion that all major inventions have been invented, all important discoveries discovered, and that we are on the threshold of understanding the secret of life and assuming control of human destiny. First it was molecules, which were supposed to be the ultimate building blocks of matter. Then came "indestructible" atoms—until protons, neutrons, and electrons were discovered. But now physicists say that all of these, too, are made up of still smaller "particles" called baryons, leptons, and mesons. There seems to be no end as ever more powerful and expensive supercolliders yield showers of finer, more primordial "quarks" and "gluons." It has been suggested that there may be as many as twenty-six dimensions of existence instead of the three or four with which we are familiar. In view of all this, a few physicists have begun to question the sanity of schemes being concocted to help us understand physical reality on both a subatomic and a cosmic level.

We may find ourselves in a similar situation when the spectral extremes of medicine are extended far beyond "ultrabirth" and "infradeath" into a comparably uncharted realm of "biological quarks" —and beyond—in order to glean a bit of knowledge of what life and death really are. It could take eons, and may never be possible. But the prospect of impossibility should not dissuade any scientist or doctor who is sincerely dedicated to the pursuit of empirical truth.

A prerequisite for that noble aim is the ideal of unfettered experimentation on human death under impeccably ethical conditions. Obitiatry, as I have outlined it, comes closest to that ideal, now and for the foreseeable future. The practice should be legitimized and implemented as soon as possible; but that calls for the strident advocacy of influential personalities who, unfortunately, choose to remain silent or disinterested—or simply antithetical.

My lone voice cannot accomplish much. But in having written this book and taken action through the practice of medicide as the first step in the right direction, I have done all that I can possibly do on behalf of a just cause for our species. I have no delusions about the end result of it all. If the lessons of history are still valid, then my evanescent proposal will quickly disappear in the infinity of time, only to be revived every millenium or two by some naive individual whose delight in having such a beneficial "original" idea inevitably will give way to the despair of futility in trying to promulgate it. By comparison, my despair will have been mild and short-lived.

But who knows—there's always the chance that some unexpected quirk of human nature will compel a generally misguided society to add a new twist to the lessons of history by doing the right thing (for a change) at the right time and instituting obitiatry without qualms and without delay.

Who knows?

References

1. Edelstein, L. "Die Geschichte der Sektion in der Antike." In *Quellen und Studien zur Geschichte der Naturwissenschaften und der Medizin*, vol. 3, pp. 50–106. Berlin: Springer-Verlag, 1932.
2. Kevorkian, J. "Medicine, Ethics, and Execution by Lethal Injection." *Medicine and Law* 4 (1985):307–13.
3. ———. "Opinions on Capital Punishment, Executions, and Medical Science." *Medicine and Law* 4 (1985):515–33.
4. ———."A Comprehensive Bioethical Code for Medical Exploitation of Humans Facing Imminent and Unavoidable Death." *Medicine and Law* 5 (1986):181–97.
5. ———."The Last Fearsome Taboo: Medical Aspects of Planned Death." *Medicine and Law* 8 (1988):1–15.
6. Walker, P. N. *Punishment: An Illustrated History*. Newton Abbot, England: David & Charles, 1972.
7. Mannix, D. P. *Those About to Die*. New York: Ballantine Books, 1958, p. 36.
8. Held, R. *Inquisition*. Florence: Qua d'Arno, 1985.
9. Andrews, W. *Old-Time Punishments*. Detroit: Singing Tree, 1970.
10. Scott, G. R. *The History of Capital Punishment*. London: Torchstream, 1953.
11. Bishop, G. V. *Executions: The Legal Ways of Death*. Los Angeles: Sherbourne, 1965.

12. Mann, G. "Schinderhannes, Galvanismus und die experimentelle Medizin in Mainz um 1800." *Medizinhistorisches Journal* 12 (1977):21–80.
13. Douglas, W. O. *Strange Lands and Friendly People.* New York: Harper & Brothers, 1951, pp. 107–108.
14. Perry, P. "Brushes with Death." *Psychology Today* (September 1988):14–17.
15. Carrell, S. "Execution Controversy Faces Physician." *American Medical News* (January 21, 1983):37–38.
16. Forssmann, W. *Experiments on Myself: Memoirs of a Surgeon in Germany.* New York: St. Martin's, 1972, pp. 75–99.
17. Malone, P. "Death Row and the Medical Model." *Hastings Center Report* 9 (October 1979):5–6.
18. Fishbein, M. *A History of the American Medical Association 1847–1947.* Philadelphia: W. B. Saunders, 1947, pp. 39, 149, 218, 438.
19. Cancila, C. "Debate Heats Up on Lethal Injection Issue." *American Medical News* (October 28, 1983):41.
20. *Euthanasia of Dogs and Cats Using Sodium Pentobarbital.* Washington, D.C.: The Humane Society of the United States, 1981, p. 6.
21. Grey, T. C., Sweeney, E. S., Wishart, D. L. "Physicians and the Death Penalty." (letters) *Western Journal of Medicine* 147 (1987):207.
22. Council on Ethical and Judicial Affairs: Recent Opinions of the Council. *Journal of the American Medical Association* 256 (1986):2241.
23. American College of Physicians Ethics Manual. Part I: "History of Medical Ethics, the Physician and the Patient, the Physician's Relationship to Other Physicians, the Physician and Society." *Annals of Internal Medicine* 101 (1984):129–37.
24. Devlin, M. M. "Execution by Lethal Injection and the Role of the Physician." *Journal of the American Medical Association* 248 (1982):3031.
25. Savage, R. "Re-paying Society." *Macon (Georgia) Telegraph and News* (February 19, 1989):E1.
26. Meredith, J. H. "Organ Procurement from the Executed." *Transplantation Proceedings* 18 (1986):406–407.
27. Al-Khadar, A. A., et al. "Renal Transplantation from HBsAg Positive Donors to HBsAg Negative Recipients." *British Medical Journal* 297 (1988):854.
28. Pappworth, M. H. *Human Guinea Pigs: Experimentation on Man.* Boston: Beacon Press, 1967.
29. Relman, A. S. "Medical Journal: A Second Opinion." (letter) *Wall Street Journal* (March 31, 1986):19.
30. Farmer, D. F. "Transfusions of Cadaver Blood: A Contribution to the

History of Blood Transfusions." *Bulletin of the American Association of Blood Banks* 13 (1960):229–34.

31. Kevorkian, J. "A Brief History of Experimentation on Condemned and Executed Humans." *Journal of the National Medical Association* 77 (1985):215–26.

32. Major, R. H. *A History of Medicine.* Springfield, Ill.: C. C. Thomas, 1954, pp. 115–51.

33. Khachigyan, L. "Anatomic Dissection in Ancient Armenia." *Bulletin of the Academy of Sciences of the Armenian Soviet Socialist Republic* No. 49 (1947):83–90.

34. Grigoryan, G. "New Evidence Proving the Existence of Dissection in the Middle Ages." *Report of the Nation Library (Soviet Armenia)* No. 6 (1962):293–96.

35. Aintabyan, P. "New Evidence with Regard to Vivisection Performed in Medieval Armenia." *Sion* 3 (1977):61–64.

36. Debus, A. G. (ed.) *World Who's Who in Science.* Chicago: Marquis-Who's Who, Inc., 1968, p. 463.

37. Rayer, P. *Traité des Maladies des Reins.* Paris: J. B. Baillière, 1841, pp. 213–14.

38. Choulant, L. *Geschichte und Bibliographie der anatomischen Abbildung.* Leipzig: Rudolph Weigel, 1852, p. 28.

39. Silverberg, R. *The Great Doctors.* New York: G. P. Putnam's Sons, 1964, p. 47.

40. Garrison, F. H. *An Introduction to the History of Medicine,* 4th ed. Philadelphia: W. B. Saunders, 1929, pp. 219–23.

41. Falloppii, G. *Medici Nostre Tempestate Clarissimi. Libelli Duo: Alter de Tumoribus Praeter Naturam.* Venetijs: Donatum Bertellum, 1563, p. 48.

42. Astruc, J. *De Morbis Venereis.* vol. 2, Napoli: Gerardi L. B. van Swieten, 1768, p. 143.

43. Kobler, J. *The Reluctant Surgeon: A Biography of John Hunter.* Garden City, N.Y.: Doubleday & Co., 1960, p. 69.

44. Weiner, D. P. "The Real Doctor Guillotin." *Journal of the American Medical Association* 220 (1972):85–89.

45. Aldini, J. *An Account of the Late Improvements in Galvanism.* London: Cuthell and Martin, 1803, pp. 189–216.

46. Hufeland, C. W. "Cabinetsschreiben Sr. Majestät des Königs von Preussen." *Neues Journal der praktischen Arzneykunde* 17 (1803):5–29.

47. Kant, I. "Rechtslehre." In W. Hastie *The Philosophy of Law.* Edinburgh: T & T Clark, 1887, p. 196.

48. Bernard, C. *An Introduction to the Study of Experimental Medicine.* New York: Henry Schuman, 1949, pp. 100–102.
49. Glaser, H. *The Drama of Medicine.* London: Lutterworth Press, 1962, p. 20.
50. Davaine, C. *Traité des Entozoaires.* Paris: J. B. Baillière, 1860, pp. xxvii–xxviii.
51. Denecke, T., and Adam, H. "Beobachtungen isolierten überlebenden menschlichen Herzen." *Zeitschrift für experimentelle Pathologie und Therapie* 2 (1906):491–509.
52. Savitt, T. L. *Medicine and Slavery.* Urbana: University of Illinois Press, 1978, pp. 293–307.
53. Bouchut, E. *Atlas d'Ophthalmoscopie médicale et de Cerebroscopie.* Paris: J. B. Ballière et Fils, 1878, pp. 56–57.
54. Kevorkian, J. "The Fundus Oculi and the Determination of Death." *American Journal of Pathology* 32 (1956):253–69.
55. Strong, R. P. "Vaccinations against Plague." *Philippine Journal of Science* 1 (1906):181–90.
56. Strong, R. P., and Crowell, B. C. "The Etiology of Beriberi." *Philippine Journal of Science* 7 (1912):271–414.
57. Katz, J. *Experimentation with Human Beings.* New York: Russell Sage Foundation, 1972, pp. 299–306.
58. Westacott, E. *A Century of Vivisection and Anti-vivisection.* Ashingdon, England: C. W. Daniel, 1949, pp. 496–501.
59. Lord, P. H. "Public Guinea Pig No. 1." *Scribner's Commentator* (March 1940):94–98.
60. Dadrian, V. N. "The Role of Turkish Physicians in the World War I Genocide of Ottoman Armenians." In *Holocaust and Genocide Studies,* vol. 1, No. 2, Oxford: Pergamon Press, 1986, pp. 169–92.
61. Lifton, R. J. "Medicalized Killing in Auschwitz." *Psychiatry* 45 (1982):283–97.
62. Alexander, L. "Medical Science under Dictatorship." *New England Journal of Medicine* 241 (1949):39–47.
63. Mitscherlich, A., and Mielke, F. *Doctors of Infamy.* New York: Henry Schuman, 1949, pp. 96, 147.
64. Edelstein, L. *The Hippocratic Oath: Text, Translation, and Interpretation.* Baltimore: Johns Hopkins Press, 1943, pp. 6–18, 38, 50–54.
65. Black, H. C. *Black's Law Dictionary,* 5th ed. St. Paul, Minn.: West Publishing Co., 1979, pp. 918–19.
66. Saint Augustine. *The City of God against the Pagans.* Cambridge: Harvard University Press, 1966, bk. 1, ch. xxi, pp. 95–96.

67. Fletcher, J. *Humanhood: Essays in Biomedical Ethics.* Buffalo, N.Y.: Prometheus Books, 1979, pp. 2–4, 46, 103, 135, 173–175, 194–198.
68. Hill, D., and Evans, D. W. "Heart and Brain Transplants." *British Medical Journal* 297 (1988):1475.
69. Kolff, J., et al. "The Artificial Heart in Humans." *Journal of Thoracic and Cardiovascular Surgery* 87 (1984):825–31.
70. Anonymous and untitled. *Hastings Center Report* (April 1986):48.
71. Ricks, D. "Pig Hearts Could Beat in Humans." *Detroit Free Press,* (12 February 1991):20.
72. Hippocrates. "Of the Epidemics, and The Law." In *Ancient Medicine and Other Treatises.* Chicago: Henry Regnery, 1949, pp. 121–23.
73. McCuen, G. E., and Boucher, T. *Terminating Life.* Hudson, Wisc.: Gary McCuen, 1985, p. 60.
74. Jones, J. H. *Bad Blood.* New York: The Free Press, 1981.
75. Langer, E. "Human Experimentation: Cancer Studies at Sloan-Kettering Stir Public Debate on Medical Ethics." *Science* 143 (1964):551–53.
76. Beecher, H. K. "Ethics and Clinical Research." *New England Journal of Medicine* 274 (1966):1354–60.
77. Anonymous. "Senile Seniors Used as Guinea Pigs." *Press-Telegram,* Long Beach, Calif. (14 May 1985):A6.
78. Hamblin, T. J. "A Shocking American Report with Lessons for All." *British Medical Journal* 295 (1987):73.
79. Seidelman, W. E. "Mengele Medicus: Medicine's Nazi Heritage." *The Milbank Quarterly* 66 (1988):221–39.
80. Carmi, A. (ed.) *Euthanasia.* Berlin: Springer-Verlag, 1984, pp. 24, 170.
81. Kevorkian, J. "The Long Overdue Medical Specialty: Bioethiatrics." *Journal of the National Medical Association* 78 (1986):1057–60.
82. Einstein, A. *Ideas and Opinions.* New York: Bonanza Books, 1954, pp. 39, 40, 104.
83. Sanger, M. *My Fight for Birth Control.* New York: Farrar & Rinehart, 1931.
84. Sumner, W. G. *Folkways: A Study of the Sociological Importance of Usages, Manners, Customs, Mores, and Morals.* New York: Dover, 1959, p. 402.
85. Cardozo, B. N. *The Growth of the Law.* New Haven: Yale University Press, 1924, pp. ix–xi.
86. Packard, H. L.: *The Limits of the Criminal Sanction.* Stanford, Calif.: Stanford University Press, 1968, p. 359.
87. Krantz, S. *Supplement to the Law of Corrections and Prisoners' Rights.* Sec. 2, chap. 6. St. Paul, Minn.: West Publishing Co., 1977, p. 28.

88. Quill, T. E. "Death with Dignity: A Case of Individual Decision Making." *New England Journal of Medicine* 324 (1991):691-94.
89. Gorowitz, S. *Doctors' Dilemmas.* New York: Macmillan, 1982, p. 218.
90. Anonymous. "Twain Pleaded for Death." *The Detroit News* (10 November 1988):1.
91. Nimmo, W. P. *Clergymen and Doctors: Curious Facts and Characteristic Sketches.* Philadelphia: J. B. Lippincott, (no date), p. 37.
92. Cant, G. "Deciding When Death Is Better than Life." *Time* (16 July 1973):37.
93. Watson, W. "The Death of George V." *History Today* 36 (December 1986):21-30.
94. Harper, T. "Where Euthanasia Is a Way of Life." *Medical Economics* (23 November 1987):23-28.
95. Cooke, P. "The Gentle Death." *Hippocrates* 3 (September/October 1989):50-60.
96. Anonymous. "MD Found Dead; Charged with Giving Overdose to Terminally Ill Friend." *American Medical News* (27 September 1985):8.
97. *People* vs *Campbell*, 1983, 335 NW Second 27, 124 Mich. App. 333.
98. Weinreb, L. L. *Criminal Law: Cases, Comments, Questions.* 2nd ed. Mineola, N.Y.: Foundation Press, 1975, pp. 291-93.
99. Adams, G. "Death, by Appointment Only. Medical Management of Death." *Health Care Weekly Review* (Detroit) [24 August 1987]:1.
100. Wanzer, S. H., et al. "The Physician's Responsibility Toward Hopelessly Ill Patients." *New England Journal of Medicine* 320 (1989):844-49.
101. Koseff, D. *The Voices of Masada.* New York: St. Martin's Press, 1973, pp. 231-37.
102. Hopfe, L. M. *Religions of the World.* 3rd ed. New York: Macmillan, 1983, pp. 276-78.
103. Tolchin, M. "Suicide Rate among Elderly Up Sharply in 80s, U.S. Finds." *The Detroit Free Press* (19 July 1989):6A.
104. Williams, G. "Euthanasia and the Physician." In M. Kohl (ed.) *Beneficent Euthanasia.* Buffalo, N.Y.: Prometheus, pp. 157-62.
105. Cutter, F. *Art and the Wish to Die.* Chicago: Nelson-Hall, 1983, p. 32.
106. Binet-Sangle, C. *L'Art de Mourir.* Paris: Albin Michel, 1919, pp. 107-52.
107. *Federal Register* 50, no. 154 (8 August 1975):33520.
108. Goodhart, C. B. "Embryo Experiments." *British Medical Journal* 297 (1988):782-83.

109. Anonymous. "It's Over, Debbie." *Journal of the American Medical Association* 259 (1988):272.
110. Kevorkian, J., and Bylsma, G. "Transfusion of Portmortem Human Blood." *American Journal of Clinical Pathology* 35 (1961):413–19.
111. Kevorkian, J., Nicol, N., and Rea, E. "Direct Body-Body Human Cadaver Blood Transfusion." *Military Medicine* 129 (1964):24–27.

Appendix

The following model code is reproduced with permission from the editor of *Medicine and Law* (see reference 4). It delineates proper conduct for any professional or lay individual in any way participating in experimentation on human beings facing undeniably imminent and inevitable death in any communal milieu which acknowledges the practice to be legal according to international standards of jurisprudence. Asterisks (*) indicate additions to the model as originally published.

(A) Any person of majority age may participate in experimentation, provided that he or she is not and never has been judged to be insane or mentally incompetent, censured for moral turpitude, convicted of any felony, or imprisoned for any reason under laws of a democratic regime.

   1. An experimenter must not take part in soliciting or in deciding on the mandate for experimentation.

   2. An experimenter may offer consultation requested by those responsible for securing such a mandate.

   3. The mandate may apply to the following prospective subjects:

      a. Condemned to death by law.

      b. Condemned to death by secular or religious canon.

      c. Condemned to imminent death by advanced disease, severe disability or trauma, or advanced senility.

      d. Condemned to death by justifiable human volition.

253

4. An experimenter must not deal with administrative matters. His (or her*) only responsibility is to select, organize, prepare for, perform, and document results of medical experiments.

(B) Administrative officials must obtain uncoerced and unwavering consent, certified in writing in the immediate witnessing presence of at least one member in good standing from each of the legal and clerical professions, directly from a prospective subject adjudged to be mentally competent, and indirectly from the legal proxy if the prospective subject is declared officially to be mentally incompetent.

1. Those responsible for obtaining consent must avoid comments beyond what is essential for the prospective subject to arrive at a reasoned decision; the former must avoid words and actions which could be construed to be unduly persuasive.

   a. A prospective subject's firm negative response eliminates him (or her*) forever from further consideration.

   b. A prospective subject's firm positive response may be reversed at will until one week prior to the scheduled date of experimentation, and his (or her*) reversal to negative eliminates him (or her*) from further consideration.

   c. Any prospective subject's firm positive response entitles him (or her*) to expert consultation from competent and reputable physicians, attorneys, theologians, psychologists, sociologists, penologists.

   d. Vacillation or uncertainty in deciding will be construed as a firm negative response.

(C) An experimenter may perform alone or as one of a heterogeneous group of physicians, other scientists, or trained laymen; a solo experimenter may be assisted by untrained laymen at his (or her*) own discretion.

1. The prospective subject has priority of choice as to the general type of research to be conducted (e.g., surgical, medical, or pharmaceutical) or the specific body parts or systems to be investigated.(*)

2. Experiments may be of any kind or complexity.

   a. Considerations of monetary funding or of personal inconvenience must not deter the undertaking of some kind of experiment, no matter how simple.

3. While a prospective subject is fully conscious, an experimenter may start any procedure which on thorough analysis portends no significant distress for the subject, and to which the investi-

gator would not hesitate to submit if he (or she*) were in identical circumstances.

   a. The procedure may be discontinued at any time by either the conscious subject or the experimenter; any subsequent action must be taken only when the subject is under surgical depth anesthesia.

   b. At the first sign or symptom of incipient distress in the subject, anesthetic resources immediately at hand must be used as soon as possible to render the subject unconscious.

     (i) Experimentation may continue only if the subject remains at or deeper than stage III general anesthesia.

     (ii) Experimentation may continue until completed or until the subject's biological death ensues.

4. Induction and irreversible maintenance of at least stage III general anesthesia is imperative before experimentation is begun on the following prospective subjects:

   a. All brain-dead, comatose, mentally incompetent, or otherwise completely uncommunicative individuals.

   b. All neonates, infants, and children less than (—) years old (age must be arbitrarily set by consensus).

   c. All living intrauterine and aborted or delivered fetuses.

5. All phases of experimentation must be carried out in the immediate presence of one or more certified, competent, and reputable witnesses representing the following societal elements:

   a. The medical and nursing professions.

   b. The judiciary or legal profession.

   c. The clergy.

   d. The administrative staff of the host institution or facility where the experiment is being performed.

   e. The prison population at large if the subject is a judicially condemned criminal.

6. If the subject's body is alive at the end of the experimentation, final biologic death may be induced by means of

   a. Removal of organs for transplantation.

   b. A lethal dose of a new or untested drug, to be administered by an official lay executioner.

   c. A lethal intravenous bolus of thiopental solution, injected by an official lay executioner.

7. No member of a research team must expect, demand, or receive remuneration, compensation, or perquisite of any kind for having participated in any way in any phase of experimentation or in the publication of results thereof.

(D) Both positive and negative results of every experiment must be disclosed fully and publicly as soon as possible.

1. Results must be published only in media devoted exclusively and entirely to any and all aspects of terminal human experimentation as outlined.

   a. The media must eschew extraneous advertisements.

   b. Editors, their associates, and authors should serve without expectation of any kind of remuneration.

2. Published reports may disclose only names, titles and addresses of authors at their discretion; and names and location of sites of experimentation.

3. Published reports must not disclose the identity of any subject of experimentation except for the following:

   a. A very brief dedicatory statement at the beginning or end of published reports may cite only the full names of immediate victims of capital crime committed by judicially condemned experimental subjects.

4. Published reports must not mention the source of funds used to support or make possible the experimentation.

As we, the condemned population of San Quentin, know, there is a
new method that could be used to execute the condemned person
called "Lethal Injection".

A person that is executed by this method would be able to donate
any part of his body to people that would live if he did this.

A person that is executed by "Lethal Gas" would not be able to
donate any part of his body to help save another.
* *
If you think that the condemned person should have the right to
choose which method should be used in the event that he must be
executed please sign your name below.

5-C-1 _Michael Wayne Jennings_
5-C-2 _J. Snow_ C-65500.1 7/24/84
5-C-3 _____
5-C-4 _Gary Lee Horenson_
5-C-5 _Donald Griffin_ C-23900. 7-25-84
5-C-6 _Theodore F. Frank_ C-13300
5-C-7 _Harold R. Memro_ C-12600
5-C-8 _____
5-C-9 _R. Phillips_ C-13707
5-C-10 _L. Betcha_ C-23400
5-C-11 _Brett P. Ponsein_ C-542.00
5-C-12 _Robert C. McFain_ C-30800
5-C-13 _Michael R. Mattson_ C-15604
5-C-14 _Richard Adam Hay_ C-05348   5-C-16 _Phillip Susso_
5-C-15 _William H. Berlin_ C-44600
5-C-17 _Phillip Sixt_ 61600
5-C-18 _Robert L. Thompson_ C-78000
5-C-19 _Robert A. Harris_ Y-4655
5-C-20 _D. J. Beardslee_ C-82702
5-C-21 _Keith E. Adcox_
5-C-22 _____
5-C-23 _____
5-C-24 _Ronald E. Fuller_ C-25143 7/24/84
5-C-27 _Melvin M. Wade_ C-43200
5-C-28 _____
5-C-29 _Mike Leach_ C-19xxx
5-C-30 _Douglas Clark_ C-63000. _Douglas Clark_
5-C-31 _Robert L. Massie_ A-90159
5-C-32 _____
5-C-33 _Michael Wayne Hunter_ C-83600
5-C-34 _Michael A. Hamilton_ C-58200
5-C-35 _____
5-C-36 _Vernon R. Odle_ C-71100
5-C-37 _____

Index